SCORE

HOW TO
WIN THE GIRL OF YOUR
DREAMS

KIRA REED

Mike !
Thanks for taking a
chance on me for my first
movie "Maui Heat" — and to
your many years of friendship.
xo Kira Reed

To Bob, my poster child.

TABLE of CONTENTS

INTRODUCTION

Hi guys! It's me—Kira Reed from Playboy TV's *Sexcetera* and all those movies you like to watch. I'm not a dumpy old sex therapist or some guy who *thinks* he's got it all figured out telling you how to get your Dream Girl. I'm a savvy, successful, hot-blooded woman who's seen it all and tried most of it. I'm a straight shooter who gets right to the point and tells it like it is. After all, life's too short to read long "how-to" books—especially when it comes to your romantic future.

The ideas in my simple seven-step plan can be used at any stage of your life and in any kind of relationship. However, *SCORE* is best for those of you who are serious about having the real deal with a great lady. I mean, if you're more interested in a happy ending than happily ever after then why bother reading a book? Why not just swing by the *Horny Co-ed* chat room? It would ultimately be less work than dating an actual hot woman. Seriously, I have nothing against trying to get you laid; however, I'm also interested in helping you become the man that a woman like my hot friends and I would actually go out with—more than once.

SCORE strives to help you get a great girl to like *the real you.* It is not the same old BS about how to trick a woman into liking *the player you.* In fact those books are such nonsense that any Hot Chick worth her push-up bra can see your pathetic, poser ass getting in a cab downtown. I mean really, do you want to just play the game… or actually win the girl?

I assume we're on the same page here. You're looking to not only meet your ultimate fantasy woman, but also get her to like you, want her to have sex with you, and keep her coming back for more. If so, let's get started!

PREGAME

I have a simple theory. It takes three basic tools to attain success: *Desire, Knowledge,* and *Action.* Whether it is getting six-pack abs, closing a business deal, or landing a hot girl, **Desire + Knowledge + Action = Success.**

The good news is if you're reading this right now you're already on the right track. You have the *desire* to make a change for the better in your love life and you are open, ready, and willing.

I have my cheerleader outfit on and I'm giving you a big "Woo Hoo!"

However, do you really know what you want? Who is your Dream Girl? What is your ultimate desire? As in all aspects of life, you must set a goal if you are going to attain it. You have to know what you're shooting for in order to score. I find that to discover what it is I truly desire, I need to write it down. Yes, literally write it down—as in make a list.

Now, you may have a special someone in mind like Suzy in advertising who struts by your office in that short skirt and tight sweater just screaming "Dream Girl!" However, most of you haven't met your perfect girl yet. It's my job to help you find her. But, in order to do so, we must know who she is.

I want you to make a list of all the qualities your perfect Dream Girl possesses. Start your list with:

"I want a woman…" ("I want a woman who's hot" is not good enough.)

"I want a woman with a college degree, who's under five feet six, likes hockey, doesn't want kids, has a heart-shaped ass, loves dogs, listens to country music, is hot-tempered, likes to be spanked, cooks Italian food, enjoys mountain biking, and gives great blow jobs."

Now we are getting somewhere. You need to get really specific with your list. Hone in on your ideal. The more details you can name about your Dream Girl the better. If you have a real life girl in mind, write down the attributes about her that you do know and like:

"Red hair, blue eyes, sweet smile, freckles, perky tits…"

Then, because I assume you don't know her all that well, add to the list what you want her to be like in more specific detail:

"I want a woman who likes sci-fi movies."

"I want a woman who enjoys a good pinot noir."

"I want a woman I can take home to Mom."

"I want a woman who lets me watch football with the boys."

"I want a woman who is ticklish."

"I want a woman who is too old to be into Justin Beiber."

"I want a woman who's old enough to appreciate Bob Dylan."

"I want a woman who wears stilettos in bed."

"I want a woman who won't drive me crazy."

You get the picture.

Now, the magic number here is one hundred. I want you to write down one hundred traits your Dream Girl possesses. Be honest. Be creative. Be idealistic. I'm serious. This is not a mental list. WRITE IT DOWN. Go get a notepad and a pen.

(I'm waiting…)

If you get stuck, don't think—just write. Judging your list as you go does not help you. Nothing is too silly or too much to ask. This is your big chance to create your perfect woman. Go for it! You can't skip this step because you think it's stupid. If you think it's stupid, you need to do it even more. Remember: be careful what you wish for because, with the help of this book, you will most likely get it. When you reach one hundred you may read on. Until then, keep writing.

OK. This is me in my cheerleading outfit giving you a big "Yea You!"

You've got a goal now. You know who she is, what kind of girl you desire. The Hot Chick hunt is well underway. You have a real shot now because you've put it out in the Universe. Now, take the list and stash it somewhere private. Don't break it out and study it. Don't edit or second-guess your list just yet. Simply leave it alone. Over the course of the book, I will ask you to revisit it. But for now—let it be.

Step 1: KNOW YOU'VE GOT A SHOT

Madonna: "Hello Garth."

Garth: "Oh my God—it's Madonna! I'm not worthy! I'm not worthy!"

Wayne: "OK OK—Garth—we're in Madonna's bedroom... Whoa!"

BOTH: "We're not worthy! We're not worthy!"

Madonna: "Shut-up—you're both worthy."

– Classic Saturday Night Live "Wayne's World" Sketch

Does the following sound like the ongoing soundtrack in your head?

"I'm not cool enough, so that hot girl won't like me."

"I'm not good looking enough, so she won't go out with me."

"I'm not rich enough, so I'm not worthy."

If this is your attitude, then you're probably miserable and alone on a Saturday night. You need to get over yourself! All that negative thinking is not getting you anywhere. So forget about it. It's time to stop with the "poor me" and "I can't" obstacles that are getting in the way of you getting your girl. Shut up already. You're worthy! There are some widely believed myths out there that are just not true. So let's lose them once and for all.

Myth #1

Everyone must be after the girl I like; therefore, I have no chance in hell.

Wrong. One of the reasons I wanted you to make a list is to realize that it's pretty damn close to impossible that any two guys in the world are going to have the exact same Dream Girl. That's because:

No one has the same ideal of a Hot Chick.

This is a good thing! Not everyone is after your perfect woman. Just you. She may be too short for that guy, or too curvy for him over there, or too smart, too funky, too serious, too blond, too wild, or too whatever for the next dude. However, if you like her, that's all that matters. You've narrowed the playing field just by focusing in on who you really want. You're already more advanced than most guys out there aimlessly gathering as many phone numbers as possible, without ever really getting anywhere near the woman who will actually make them happy. You are already head and shoulders above the competition, so get over the idea that you have no chance in hell. You do!

Myth #2

I'm not hot; therefore, I can't score a Hot Chick.

Wrong again, Buddy. Let me fill you in on a little secret:

Hot Chicks like being the center of attention.

Pretty, savvy women like being the one that everyone in the room notices as she makes an entrance. Good-looking women are vain, insecure, and in need of approval. As long as they have the spotlight where they want it (on themselves), they're happy. But, if the guy she's with is the one that everyone in the room looks at with wanton eyes, *she's jealous.* It's true. I'm not lying. Most attractive women I know want to be the hot one in the couple. If people are staring at the guy, a woman wants it to be because *they wish they had her*, not because *they wish to look like him.*

As most of you know, I am happily married to a wonderful man. Now, don't get me wrong. I find my husband very attractive. However, on first look, some might say he's *chubby, balding, hairy, and short.*

Yes. He actually is all of those things. He also happens to be *kind, generous, and smart.*

He is a great joke teller.

He does yoga.

He loves animals.

He enjoys live music.

He travels to fun places.

He knows wine.

He opens the door for me.

He smells good.

He puts up with my shit.

He dresses impeccably.

He's a great problem solver.

... and he eats fantastic pussy.

All of which are on my Perfect Man list.

Therefore, my man is super-sexy *to me*. To tell you the truth, I'm glad he doesn't look like Brad Pitt. Otherwise, I'd spend my whole life beating women off with a stick, and no one would ever pay attention to *me*. So get over the idea you can't get a Hot Chick. It's a lie. You can!

Myth # 3

She must already be taken; therefore, I shouldn't ask her out.

Here's something that you must understand:

If she isn't wearing a ring, she's available.

Seriously. Does she have a big rock or a wedding band on her left hand? If she doesn't have a ring, chances are she wants to be asked out. Also, more good news here: the hotter the chick, the less likely it is she has a date this weekend. Why? Because she's so dynamic and gorgeous she intimidates men. It takes balls to approach a beautiful, mysterious stranger and ask her to go eat food with you.

Now, most guys are doing the same thing you've been doing without success: assuming "everyone is after her" (Myth #1), thinking "she's hot and I'm not" so she will say no (Myth #2), then deducing that "she's unavailable" (Myth # 3). It takes a courageous man to walk up to a woman, make conversation, and ask for a date. FYI: We hot women find courage a turn-on!

The fact of the matter is Hot Chicks are not asked out enough because guys are scared and don't realize that:

She is highly likely to say "yes."

A woman will say "yes" for any number of reasons—all of which are good for you because they give you a shot with this girl. She will say "yes" to a date with you:

Because you smell good (learn more in Step 2).

Because you dress well (learn more in Step 3).

Because she thinks you're kinda cute.

Because you're the complete opposite of her last boyfriend.

Because she doesn't want to be alone this Saturday either.

Because it's been a long time since she's gotten laid and she's horny.

Because she is looking for her perfect man too… and you just might be him.

Who cares why? At least you've got her where you want her—with you. The rest will come with a little help from this book.

Even if she's not available, an attractive woman will be thrilled that you asked her out on a date. She won't think you're a loser for asking even if she says "no." Believe me. I've been there and *all* my hot girlfriends agree. Not only will she be flattered, she will probably regret having to turn you down because she's in a so-so relationship and *you* may be her last hope of somebody better than the loser boyfriend she's been shacking up with. Even if she says "no" to a date with you because she is currently seeing someone, you never know what the future may hold. Some day she may be free from her current relationship and know that you're interested because you had the courage to ask. For example, this happened to me…

An oddly attractive kid approached me at a café in my neighborhood. I call him "kid" because he was a few years my junior. He was a tall, scrawny, grad student/ guitar player who was too cool for school. Let's call him

Alex. I was nice to him but not overly flirtatious as I was seeing someone at that time. After a few gallant attempts of making small talk, Alex asked me if I'd like to go out sometime. I told him thanks but I couldn't because I was in a relationship. He was a little embarrassed, but sweetly so, and we basically said, "See ya around." There were no hard feelings when we bumped into each other over the next few months at local spots as we went about our separate lives.

Cut to five months later. I am sitting alone at my favorite dive bar nursing a pint while lamenting the mistakes of my final—no really *final*—breakup with my on-again, off-again boyfriend, when lo and behold Alex bellies up. We got to chatting; he bought the next round and asked about "the boyfriend." When I tell him we are no longer together, he smiles and pops the question again: "So you wanna go out sometime? My buddy just opened up a new restaurant." I said "yes," we agreed on a date, and he got my number; we went to his friend's funky vegan hole-in-the-wall joint and had a great time. We ended up seeing each other for a few very fun months of raunchy sex, organic pasta, and me being groupie to his kick-ass hipster rock band. While it was not my end-all be-all relationship, Alex went off to India to find himself (I already knew who I was), it was a positive experience because he was patient and persistent in asking me out and we had some good times. So, get over the idea she's taken because she probably isn't or won't always be.

Myth #4

She's too good for me; therefore, I don't deserve her.

This is the silliest thing I've ever heard. Why would you sabotage your desire to be with an amazing woman with: "She's too *whatever* for me." For example:

"She's *too pretty to go out with me.*"

"She's too stylish to like me."

"She's too sophisticated for me."

"She's too smart to be into me."

"She's too sexy to be attracted to me."

I mean, how can a woman be *too anything good*?

What you really mean is that you don't think you are worthy of the woman you are attracted to. Believing this myth is simply counteractive to your goal. It makes no logical sense that you don't deserve what you desire. It is your inalienable right to pursue life, liberty, and the pursuit of happiness with your Dream Girl. Buck up, man, and get over it, or you will never be worthy. We hot women can smell pathetic self-doubt from a mile away. You can't hide it with a boatload of Paco Rabanne. Unworthiness is simply a turn-off. If you believe you are not good enough, we will not want to talk to you, go out with you, or have sex with you.

I'm a great guy and deserve a great woman. This should be the mantra in your head at all times when you are trying to attract a woman. Now, I'm not saying all you have to do is believe in yourself and visualize your Dream Girl and the law of attraction will magically make your über-babe appear. I'm simply saying that believing that you are *deserving* of happiness with a wonderful woman is a good place to start. We've all done stupid shit in our lives that we regret or we have something about ourselves that we wish we could change. Nevertheless, you need to forgive yourself and like who you are before you can get anyone else to like you back.

I'm a great guy and I deserve a great woman.

Say it out loud in the mirror ten times before you leave the house every day, before you go to sleep at night, and before you ask that cute hostess from the sushi place out on a date with you. I know. You're probably thinking, "This is ridiculous." It's not! The positive message you give yourself will help get rid of any negative vibe and give you the air of confidence that a girl like me and my Hot Chick friends would actually want to go out with. Come on. What harm can it do? After all, a guy should do anything that'll help get him laid.

Just so you know, all the women out there that you want to be dating are going through the same thing you are. They're getting up every morning to a cruel and competitive world, putting on a game face, and overcoming all their own issues. Even the hottest of women have their own "mishegoss" to overcome like shyness, a recent breakup, or fear of not being pretty, thin, young, smart, sexy, stylish or whatever-enough *for a great guy like you.* Yes, even the seemingly perfect, put-together women have worthiness issues. We're just as full of shit as you are. So get over the idea she's too good for you. You deserve her. You deserve each other.

Myth # 5

I don't have money; therefore, she won't go out with me.

It's true: we are living in a material world and I am a Material Girl. I cannot argue with the fact that almost all of the hot women I know, myself included, expect the man to pick up the check on a date. If you want to split the tab, she will most likely split on you. To date any woman, let alone a "ten," you need enough money in your pocket to pay the waiter. However, you don't need to be Sugar Daddy Warbucks to score a hot babe. As long as you can take care of yourself, pay your rent, not borrow money from us, have enough cash to spend on simple things like dinner and a movie, and have some extra dough to occasionally drop on small, thoughtful gifts like music, flowers, or perfume, you are indeed dating material.

If you are borderline broke, you will need to make up for your lack of cash in other ways. It can be done. In fact, there is a category of men that my girlfriends and I have dubbed *Sexy Poor.* These attractive, starving artist types include poets, musicians, eco-activists, yoga masters, or other "less-is-more" kind of alternative lifestyle poor. If this is the case, you must acknowledge us as your muse by painting our portrait, writing songs about us, drawing our bath, and giving us frequent foot massages. You must also be generous in bed and generally worship the ground we walk on. Otherwise, we won't put up with the fact that you have a roommate when you're thirty and/or sleep on a mattress on the floor. Whether you are a future business mogul in the making who is still delivering pizza or a laid-off insurance executive making ends meet by selling appliances at Best Buy, the good news is it's easier than ever before to pull off *Sexy Poor.* You used to have to drive a cool car to pick up a Hot Chick. Now you can tell her you ride a bike "for the environment."

Regardless of your profession, you can be struggling financially and still be attractive to a woman as long as you have *passion* and *potential.* This means you must *be talented* in your field of choice and *be working your ass off* to be successful. Lazy and poor do not mix. You might not land a lady that likes to go to trendy restaurants, expects gifts of designer handbags, and dreams of a five-carat diamond engagement ring by being a talented, ambitious, yet struggling... novelist. However, that kind of woman is too crude and shallow to be your Dream Girl anyway. Even with a limited bank account, if you follow the instructions I give you in the chapters to come, plenty of hot women will find you attractive. You may not score any gold diggers, mind you, but that's a good thing. So get over the idea you need big bucks to score a Hot Chick. You don't!

Bottom Line: You don't have to be George Clooney to score a "ten."

Step 2: CLEAN-UP YOUR ACT

Your shower shoes have fungus on them. You'll never make it to the bigs with fungus on your shower shoes. Think classy, you'll be classy. If you win 20 in the show, you can let the fungus grow back on your shower shoes and the press'll think you're colorful. Until you win 20 in the show, however, it means you are a slob. – Crash Davis (Kevin Costner) in *Bull Durham*

Crash is a very smart man. I speak for all women when I say I may eventually find it cute when you wear your smelly, stained Pink Floyd concert T-shirt around the house all day and skip shaving for a week. But, until you actually win me with your seductive scent, impeccable style, and soft kissable skin, you're just a bum. Cleanliness is key when trying to score a hot babe.

Note: If you haven't seen *Bull Durham*, go online and download it from Netflix right now. It's a poetic movie starring Kevin Costner, Susan Sarandon, and Tim Robbins about sex and baseball and the pursuit of happiness. A must see.

Now, you may not think you need to read this if you are a neat freak or an immaculately groomed perfectionist. However, most of you could use a refresher course from a woman's point of view. These are a few things that all women notice that are immediate turn-offs, and anyone who possesses the following bad hygiene traits is what we hot women call a *Dirty Bird*.

Dirty Bird. Noun. Definition: 1. A man who smells ripe, needs to change his shirt, is covered in "mystery film," has bad breath, and doesn't wash his hands. 2. May believe oneself to be Jim Morrison or Charles Bukowski reincarnate. 3. Slang for smelly, messy, no-ambition loser. 4. aka: not dating material. To be sure you're not harboring any *Dirty Bird* tendencies or any other lifestyle habits that are turn-offs to your potential Dream Girl, avoid these Dirty No-Nos.

Dirty Scent

Men tend to be stimulated visually… Nice hair, big tits, long legs = Hot. Women are more scent-oriented. An instant turn-off for a girl is a man with a bad body odor. This could be from not showering, not using deodorant, or wearing a pair of socks or underwear for more than one day. Too much cologne is also a turn-off. It overpowers your natural attractive scent and only masks bad hygiene. There is a difference between smelling good and smelling up the room with your aftershave. Foul body odor or strong perfumes are an assault on our sensitive sense of smell and we won't want to get near you. Once you've attracted her with your subtle scent and are actually dating her, you can run your collection of aftershaves by her to see what she likes best. Or, pick one out together that makes her want to jump you.

Goal: Get clean and fresh so she will want to get closer.

Dirty Skin

The skin is the largest organ of your body. You may think something else is—but that's just a guy thing. Clean, soft skin that we want to rub our bodies up against is key in attracting an über-babe. Wash your face. Get an exfoliating cleanser if you have clogged pores or oily skin. Blackheads on your face will send her running in the opposite direction. Even girls who have a crazy zit-popping fetish, like me, do not want to squeeze them from places you can see and reach yourself. If you have a real issue with acne, a rash, or eczema, go to a dermatologist and get help. Fast! If you have dandruff, get a dandruff shampoo from a doctor if over-the-counter doesn't do the trick. If you have dry, flaking skin, get some moisturizer. These products are not too girly—they are necessary.

Goal: Get soft skin so she will want to touch you.

Dirty Hands

We all know that we're supposed to wash our hands—I hope. Washing your hands includes washing under your nails. Your nails should be trimmed, clean, and smooth. Chewed up cuticles are not hot. Scraggly fingers and rough skin hurt—especially in our sensitive areas. Not sure what to do? Get a manicure. You'll see how to do it, and you just may like it and make it a regular good hygiene ritual. While you're at it, get a pedicure too. There is nothing worse than a man with a scary, yellow, infected toenail or dry, calloused heels. Regular use of hand and foot creams help keep away the rough edges. Do it—we'll be grateful. Believe me.

Goal: Get good hands so she will want you to touch her.

Dirty Hair

Wash your hair, guys. Greasy hair is so not sexy. It doesn't matter if you have three hairs or a full head, keep it clean and don't overload it with product. Just like you, we want to be able to run our fingers through your hair, so don't lacquer it up with spray, gel, or mousse. And for God's sake, don't attempt to spray on any hair, get plugs, create a comb-over, or wear a toupee. It's a huge turn-off. Accept the hair you have. If you are balding, trim it shorter or shave it all off. You can't fake it, so stop trying. There is a misconception out there that women think face stubble is sexy. It's not. It hurts. It rips our sensitive lady face and we won't want to kiss you. Shave. While you're at it, lose the mustache, goatee, mutton shops, and all weird patterns of hair on your face. It's not sexy; it's annoying. Don't forget to trim your eyebrows and the back of your neck. Your hairdresser can do it for you if you ask. And if you have a unibrow, fix it. Get it waxed and buy a pair of tweezers. Tweezers are your friend. There are great male grooming products out there that trim nose and ear hair. Yes, you have it. Yes, we see it. Please get rid of it. Your hair on your face isn't the only place that needs consistent attention. Please trim your pubes and shave your balls. You don't like a jungle down there and neither do we.

Goal: Get smooth so she will want to rub her face all over you.

Dirty Mouth

I'm not talking language here, though speaking like a sailor probably won't help get you a great woman. I mean your actual mouth. Success, style, and good looks don't mean a thing if she doesn't want to kiss you. Bad breath has been known to be a deal breaker. Brush your teeth, floss, and gargle mouthwash not just before bed, but before you leave the house, after you eat lunch, and of course before a big date. At the very least, keep mouth spray and mints handy and check your teeth for food remnants after eating. If your breath is chronically bad—meaning *you* can smell it or someone has mentioned it more than once—see a dentist. You may have an infection. Bad teeth are another no-no. There is nothing wrong with a bit of a crooked smile. Look at Hugh Grant or Tom Cruise. However, if your mouth is a mess, and you know who you are, fix it. Seriously. Get a recommendation from a friend if you don't have a dentist and make an appointment—today. Another good thing to do is whiten your teeth. There are whitening strips available in the drug store. It's easy and takes ten years off of your look immediately.

Goal: Get tasty fresh so she will want to taste you.

Dirty Car

I hate to sound shallow and materialistic, but let's face it: you are what you drive. Your car is an extension of you, so cleanliness is also key when it comes to your automobile. At the beginning of my acting career, when I was in my early twenties, I was going to a bunch of casting calls. My agent gave me some sage advice when she said to me, *"The audition starts when you pull up. Always keep your car clean."* The reasoning behind her statement was that if I showed up in a clean car, I would be deemed worthy, responsible, and together enough to be hired for the production. Luckily she didn't say I had to have a fancy sports car because I had a go-cart of a Volkswagen. But, I kept it immaculate and always felt perfectly respectable pulling up to wherever I was going, including swanky Hollywood hotspots. My point is do the best with what you've got. Even a zillion dollar Lamborghini will look shabby if it's loaded with fast food containers and smelly gym clothes and is covered in bird droppings. Also, if you have a crappy Honda Civic, don't try to dress it up with a spoiler and fancy rims. It only makes you look like you're trying too hard. The perfect car is a simple sedan that's comfortable and elegant. A scooter or open-air Jeep is not a real vehicle and no mode of transportation for picking up a hot babe. Neither is a monster truck. If you're in the market for a new car and don't have a lot of dough, go for a hybrid like a Toyota Prius. Girls will think you're eco-sexy for going green. I mean, if Leonardo DiCaprio drives one, so can you. Just remember to run it through the car wash before your big date.

Goal: Get a clean car to pick up dirty (in a good way) chicks.

Dirty Clothes

Do what your mother told you and wear clean underwear. Change them on *at least* a daily basis. Wash your jeans not only when you drip mustard on them but every few times you wear them, or the smokin' hot, sophisticated lady you've been ogling won't want you getting near her. Don't wear the same smelly workout clothes for a week before washing them. That's simply disgusting. Also, well-worn fashion is not the same as worn out. There's a difference between a fashionably distressed fabric and a fraying collar. Get it together to do your laundry regularly or send it to the cleaners. Throw out anything that is beyond repair or permanently stained or damaged—like those nasty shower shoes.

Goal: Get your clothes cleaned if you want to get the girl.

Dirty House

Eventually the goal is to get her back to your place. Your apartment, house, condo, or what have you doesn't have to be fancy. However, it does need to be clean. Cheese stuck in the carpet, piles of Xbox games and four-day-old dishes in the sink is not hot. It's pathetic. You won't get laid with a bachelor pad that looks like Theta Chi threw up all over it. Easy ways to start if you are knee-deep in pizza boxes is to simply TAKE OUT THE TRASH—yes, that includes the milk crates you are using as end tables. An easy way to hide the clutter that you call your "man stuff" is to get furniture that doubles as storage compartments, like trunks and coffee tables and cabinets with drawers. Also, there is a simple invention called a laundry basket. Get some wicker ones with lids, then take the wet towels and dirty shorts off the floor and put them in the basket. And, do yourself a favor and hide the girlie mags. She doesn't want to see them.

Goal: Chick Magnetize your pad so your Dream Girl will want to stay.

Dirty Fridge

Your Dream Girl also does not appreciate a dirty fridge. Crusty peanut butter jars, leftover Chinese food from God knows when, and a flat two-liter bottle of orange soda is not food—it's toxic. Get rid of the gross crap and stock your fridge with *actual food.* I am a wildcat in the bedroom; however, I hate to break it to you, but I'm like your mother in the kitchen. I have this crazy theory: you attract what you eat. If you eat healthy food that makes you look and feel good, you'll attract a healthy mate who looks and feels good too. If you eat junk food, you'll feel like shit and attract a mate who looks like a Big Mac. I know it's a bit "out there." But, I dare you to prove me wrong.

Seriously, I do know a thing or two about health and exercise. Being an actress and television host, I've always had to watch my figure. It's true the camera adds weight, so I've always had to keep mine in relative check. Out of interest in my own health and fitness, I went on to formally study and become a Certified Nutritional Counselor and yoga instructor.

Now, I'm not saying you have to be a health nut and have Hugh Jackman's abs and Ryan Reynold's arms to get a girl. However, you must attempt basic good eating habits and be moderately physically active. Guys who live on chili cheese fries and beer will not land Hot Chicks—unless they are rock stars. But if that were the case, you wouldn't be reading this book because you'd probably be getting a blow job by a barely legal groupie on your tour bus in between slices of Pizza Hut and bong hits. Since you're not Slash, I'm going to walk you through my *Seven Simple Steps Toward Good Health*.

I don't want to bore you with too many details about the acid alkaline balance or make you follow some whack-job diet where you can't eat anything but soybeans and twigs. However, whether you want to detox from your junk food diet, lose a few pounds around the middle, or simply get the healthy glow that'll attract a hot woman, here are a few no-nonsense basics. No one will care about you or your health unless you do first—well, maybe your mother, but you're not trying to get her in the sack.

Seven Simple Steps Toward Good Health

1. Don't Do Drugs

They're nasty. Toxic is not sexy. Just look what's happened to Britney Spears. And, let's not forget the ever-growing number of high-profile deaths related to prescription drugs. May MJ, Heath, Anna Nicole, Whitney and the ever-growing list of celebrity prescription drug overdoses all rest in peace. If you do take a variety of prescription drugs for whatever reason, go to mymedicalrecords.com— my genius husband's brainchild. MMR has a great drug interaction checker to keep you from inadvertently doing harm to your health by mixing drugs that don't belong together. Also, don't drink alcohol in excess. Smoking like a chimney and partying like a frat boy is not attractive; it is stupid and will scare off Hot Chicks who actually have their lives together. Avoid doing straight-up shots of anything, especially on a date. I know from experience it will only lead to disaster. And let's not forget the most import reason not to get too loaded on anything: drug and alcohol abuse will render you totally useless in bed.

2. Drink Lots of Water

Diet Coke, coffee drinks, and sugary sports-water don't count and have the opposite effect. You need a lot of fresh water to function normally, stay regular, and flush out all the junk you put in your body every day. If you need a kick to your water, try adding some lemon. It is super detoxing and fights bad breath and body odor. Lemon is extremely alkalizing and will help balance the effects of highly acidic foods like meat, coffee, alcohol, and sugar. If you like sweet, try VitaminWater Zero. (No, they don't pay me for the plug. I wish! I heard Kobe got like $100 zillion bucks or something. I just happen to really like the lemonade multivitamin one.) It's sweetened with Stevia—a natural, no-calorie substance—and chock full o' vitamins. Just don't get the regular VitaminWaters by mistake. They're 150 calories and full of sugar. Also, make it a habit to keep a water bottle on you at all times to remind yourself to stay hydrated. Drink before you get thirsty. By the time you feel the need to quench a thirst, you are already in dehydration mode.

3. Eat More Vegetables

I'm not saying starve yourself on salads. We Hot Chicks don't like it when a man eats like a girl. However, a side of asparagus or broccoli, or my favorite, spinach, is a hell of lot better for you than the double-stuffed-twice-baked potato with butter on top or the mystery-seasoned deep fried, bread-battered curly fries. I keep my fridge stocked with prewashed, ready-to-eat salad bags and cut veggies for easy no-prep meals. Just add some grilled chicken to the salad, which you can also find premade and presliced if that's your idea of cooking, and you have a no-hassle light lunch. Or, steam some veggies alongside your pizza or cheesesteak to help balance out the heavy load.

4. Don't OD on Bs: Bread, Buns, Biscuits, Bagels, etc.

White flour-based bread products are like eating paste. Choosing whole grains instead makes bread a better choice, but it still contains a boatload of carbohydrates if you don't watch your portion size. Beware of the typical predinner bread basket. I know you're hungry by the time you actually sit down to eat in a restaurant, but devouring the whole basket before your meal really starts easily spoils an otherwise healthy dinner of chicken and steamed vegetables. I understand that every once in a while a toasted New York bagel with a slab of cream cheese is a must-have. If you are going to carb load on bread, cereal, oatmeal, or a bagel, do it in the a.m. so you have the whole day to burn it off. Just know that a muffin the size of your head is a special treat, not an every morning snack. Remember: If you eat the Pillsbury dough, you'll look like the Pillsbury Doughboy.

5. Avoid Sugar

This is a tough one because sugar is hidden everywhere. It's especially hard to avoid sugar if you've got a sweet tooth like me. But I find if I go for the good stuff, a little goes a long way and I don't need as much to satisfy my sugar craving. One Godiva truffle won't kill you. But a supersize Snickers bar just might push you over the edge. I sometimes spoil myself at the end of the day with a small cup of Häagen Dazs ice cream. But I don't eat the whole pint while standing alone in the kitchen sink at two a.m.

just because I can't sleep. Things to totally avoid are high fructose corn syrup and artificially flavored and colored kid candy stuff. Stay away from anything you can buy at the checkout stand or movie theater unless you want instant diabetes. I know an apple or a banana doesn't sound that exciting, but having a piece of fruit can curb the urge for more dangerous sweets with their natural sugar. I love keeping a bunch of grapes in the refrigerator. They're way yummier than jelly beans and have actual "food value," as my mother likes to call it. With fruit, you'll still get the energy boost the candy gives you, but you'll avoid the post-sugar binge crash. If you must have something out of a wrapper, go for a nutrition bar like Quest Bars. They taste like a candy bar, but they have 20 grams of protein and only about 200 calories.

6. Eat Lean Meat

If you're like me, you enjoy a big, thick, juicy steak once in a while. But, when I do, I choose a lean filet and lay off the sauces. It's not battered, southern fried, or covered in cheese. It's also a six-ounce filet, not a slab of meat the size of a whole plate. Chicken and fish are great sources of lean protein—just not when they're breaded, deep-fried, or smothered in gravy. If you like to grill, it's the best way to go. Break out your BBQ and throw on some lean marinated steaks, chicken, or fish. You don't need to smother your meat in store-bought syrupy sauces. Simple sea salt, pepper, and a little Worcestershire go a long way.

Think about it. If you die of heart disease from all the fatty, breaded, chicken-fried steak you consume, you will not be able to live happily ever after with your dream babe.

7. Take a Good Multivitamin

Unless you know absolutely everything about orthomolecular medicine and food combining, live on a self-sustaining farm, and raise all your own organic food, you are not getting all the nutrients you need. The simplest, most effective first step toward good health is to take a high-quality multivitamin. It's the easiest thing to do. So there's no excuse not to do it. One-A-Day Men's Health Formula and Centrum's A to Zinc are available just about everywhere and are consistently rated the best of the big brands. You could also go to a health food store like Whole Foods and ask the cute hippie chick on the vitamin aisle to help you find one. If you don't like taking pills, try a nutritional supplement protein shake. I love Designs for Health's PaleoMeal. You can get them easily online. *News Flash*: Taking vitamins does not give you permission to eat garbage like fast-food. If you think you can eat fast-food and not get sick and fat and die a premature death, watch the movie *Super Size Me*.

Bonus: Get Moving

What you put into your mouth is the most important thing you can do toward good health. However, exercise is also essential if you want to land hot babes. If you work out, it shows. Run, swim, do yoga, do something! Don't just join the gym to stare at girls; actually use the machines. Workouts that include lifting weights give you good posture and broad shoulders, which, in turn, makes Hot Chicks think you're strong and manly and can protect them from the big bad world—aka a guy we'd want to go home with. You don't have to be a body builder. If fact, the no neck, no penis, overbulked look is really not sexy to most women I know. You don't even have to go to a gym to build muscle. Simply doing twenty push-ups and fifty crunches when you roll out of bed really makes a difference. Subscribe to *Men's Health* magazine or look up easy exercise routines online. Walk when you can instead of drive, like when you go for lunch three blocks away. Make time for sports you enjoy, like biking or tennis or golf. It doesn't matter what you do—just do it. Exercise gives you a healthy vibe that attracts women and gets the blood flowing to all the right places. And, yes, sex is great exercise!

Bottom Line: Clean up your act if you want to score hot women.

Step 3: PACKAGE YOURSELF

Women go crazy for a sharp dressed man. – ZZ Top

A guy has got to look sharp to be cool. I don't mean skin deep, surface, or trendy cool. I am referring to the calm, confident, collected kind of cool that comes from being comfortable in your own skin and knowing that you look good. If you package yourself well, your wardrobe will do a lot of the work of attracting ladies for you. Most women, including me, will confess that an impeccable man in a designer, slim cut suit makes them wet. It's a great look that says: Style. Success. Sex. My perfect man looks amazing dressed up. However, he also has a casual side and knows how to relax on a date. Even when he dresses down, he is always well put together because he follows my *Hot Guy Uniform Equation.*

Crisp Jeans + Dress Shirt + Fitted Sport Coat = Hot Guy.

This is the uniform for most dating occasions. If you're attending a no-jeans kind of place (not my favorite for most dates by the way), simply substitute slacks for the jeans. Yes, I understand some of you may be bikers. While steel toe boots and beer Ts are possibly an acceptable uniform for picking up chicks at dive bars, they are not appropriate for dinner for two at the cozy little bistro around the corner.

Some of you may be business executive types, so a suit and tie is your daily routine. Just don't show up for your date looking like you're trying to close a deal—or you won't. You may be into bondage in the bedroom, but nine times out of ten, if you're wearing a mesh T-shirt, latex pants, and a studded collar in public, you'll never know if she's kinky too because you'll scare her off before you can find out. All the many facets of your work, hobbies, and freaky fetishes can be explored down the road. Ultimately, your perfect girl will let you know what she likes and dislikes. But in the beginning, be a good boy, don't fight it, and dress like I tell you.

The Jeans

Dark, clean denim works for everyone. Dark colors are slimming and look more dressed up than lighter jeans. Go for a medium rise. Too-high rises will make you look like a dork. I know some guys who have a bit of a belly don't like the new lower-cut styles because they think the bulge hangs over. They're used to squeezing a belt tight to give some sort of waist. But, believe me, that looks worse than letting go a little and going with a more modern cut. I've never met a guy that can't find a nice mid-rise Joe's jean that looks fabulous. Diesel, 7 for All Mankind, and Lucky Brand are also good bets. Avoid the too tattered jeans—it looks sloppy. Ditto on the overly decorative washes and big pocket patterns. Simple, clean lines rule the denim department.

The Dress Shirt

I'm talking great fabric, tailored to fit, button-down, long-sleeved dress shirts. The kind you send to the cleaners and they come back folded in a box so you can keep a fresh one in your desk or in your car, so you will always have it handy in case of a spill or a last-minute date with a Hot Chick after work. Get a few whites and some business blues, but also try some stripes and seasonal colors. Have fun with the shirts. This is a great way to personalize your look. Go to a nice department store and get a salesperson to help you and try them on. Be sure to fit them each individually because the same shirt in a slightly different fabric will fit a bit differently. Whatever brand you choose, be sure it's soft spun cotton—no stiff stuff. Remember, the softer the fabric the more we will want to pet you.

The Sport Coat

Invest in one or two good sport coats, in a basic black, grey, or navy, and you can wear them everywhere. Fine wool that's smooth as a hot babe's bum is way sexier than that itchy polyblend number at the men's suit outlet. One spectacular sport coat in a fantastic fabric is better than a closet full of poorly structured, ill-fitting ones in cheap material. Italian designers are great for slimmer builds while American brands fit better for broader shoulders and waistlines. Be sure to avoid overly boxy cuts that make you look dated and wider and shorter than you really are.

Shopping Tip: Call the upscale department stores and sign up for their mailing lists. It's the best way to find out when they're having a sale so you can get the good stuff without breaking the bank. At least twice a year, the major stores have a forty to sixty percent off insider sale.

But wait, there's more…

The Shoes and Belt

Just like the Dude's rug "really pulled the room together," good accessories complete your look. Many people, including me, subscribe to the theory that the shoes make the man. I must admit, hot women will judge a man by what he wears on his feet. Simple, well-made brown or black leather is the way to go. Lace-ups or loafers are up to you as long as they don't look like slippers. Don't skimp. We've seen what's in the window at Payless, and that's where it should stay. Don't get too fancy, pointy, or overly exotic. You're not the girl in this scenario. Keep your shoes in good shape and looking good. All the shoeshine stations on the street are there for a reason. High-top Chuck Taylors are not acceptable footwear in the uniform. Your belt should in most cases match the shoes in color and style of leather. Unless you live in Texas, own a ranch, or are actually a real-life cowboy, oversize western belt buckles are not cool.

About Suits

The same principles apply for suits as sport coats. Simple, slimming lines in good fabrics are key. These days a suit doesn't have to be buttoned up and tied like a banker, even if you are one. If you're a corporate kinda guy, great. But take off the tie and show your lady your softer side when wining and dining and winning her over. Save the sexy suit for a special occasion like when you whisk her off to the opera al la *Pretty Woman*. FYI: Corduroy is not an acceptable fabric for a suit—unless you're Jason Schwartzman, and then maybe you can pull it off.

The Extras

A simple, elegant watch is a major plus. A solid gold Rolex is not necessary. However, a basic TAG Heuer or Cartier stainless steel sport watch says you know what time it is. Man jewelry is fun as long as it is genuinely you. A chain or an earring or a chunky bracelet is great, as long as it is actually something you like, not just something you are using to impress, like a flashy bling ring. Also, if you are not really into skulls and black diamond dog tags and piercings, you will look ridiculous trying to pull them off. Stick to accessories that accentuate who you are, not attempt to make you someone you are not. Remember, Hot Chicks like stylish men, but not total phonies.

P.S. You should carry a sleek, good condition leather wallet. No, it should not hang on a chain. Yes, if it says

Gucci on it we will probably take notice, but it is so not necessary to be a label hound. That is more of a Hot *Chick* thing to do.

P.P.S. You don't have to spend a million bucks to look like a million bucks. That's why God invented designer discount stores. I can usually find some killer buys at Loehmann's, which has a fantastic men's store.

Just in case you haven't been on a date since before the Internet was invented, here are some other looks to lose now:

Workout clothes from the Aerobics era

Tube socks. Short shorts and tucked in tank tops. Unless you are Will Ferrell, you can't pull it off. And who wants to look like Will Ferrell anyway?

T-shirts under blazers

This wannabe Don Johnson look dates you big time. Seriously, guys, *Miami Vice* was never really cool.

Things attached to you

A cell phone, keys, chain hang wallet, or whatever you have attached to your waist looks ridiculous. You don't look important or cool with your "Crackberry" attached to you. You reek geek. And, not in the *Glee* geek-chic way. You might as well wear a pocket protector while you're at it.

Do-rag

You are not Bret Michaels so get over yourself. You will never have a reality show with a bunch of bimbos girl-fighting each other to win a chance to fuck you. Seriously. Don't dress like you're a rock star—unless you are a rock star.

Monogrammed clothing

Overly monogrammed, pressed Brooks Brothers Oxford wear is not sexy. It's dorky—unless we are role-playing the preppy and the cheerleader. Then, it is super-hot.

Graphic Ts and hats

Sorry guys. Jon Gosselin, Kevin Federline, and the *Real House Husbands of New Jersey* have ruined it for all y'all. The Ed Hardy overload is OUT!

The easiest way to stay relatively current is to subscribe to a men's fashion magazine like *GQ* or *Esquire*. You don't have to look like the guy in the underwear ad, but you may like the cut of his boxer briefs…and so will she.

One More Thing

Team jerseys or other athletic logo wear are not real clothes. They are to be saved for the gym, drinking beer with your buddies, or attending sporting events—not for going out in public with hot babes.

If you follow my simple Hot Guy Uniform Equation and wear what I tell you to wear, I guarantee it will immediately boost your desirability and give you an air of confidence when you walk into any situation where you want to attract women. You will feel more secure and, therefore, more confident. However, there are still some things that need to be projected from the inside that go beyond the cut of your clothes.

Wouldn't this be a great world if insecurity and desperation made us more attractive? If "needy" were a turn-on?

– Aaron Altman (Albert Brooks) in *Broadcast News*

If you haven't seen *Broadcast News*, go get it. It's a sexy, savvy, smart relationship flick featuring Holly Hunter, Albert Books, and William Hurt and is directed by James L. Brooks. It's a great movie and Albert Brooks' character, Aaron Altman, is about as needy and desperate as you can get. Therefore, though he is the heroine's (Holly Hunter's) best friend, he is never considered potential dating material.

What is Cool?

Cool means you are a whole person, so you don't need a Hot Chick on your arm to complete you. Cool comes from letting go, not trying so hard, and just being genuinely *you*. Cool is not about superficial ego inflation like, *"I don't need anyone"* or *"I'm so great, all chicks dig me."*

That attitude is plain cocky and just as unattractive as its desperate opposite *"I can't live without her."* News Flash: If you couldn't live without her, you'd be dead already.

The best way I have found to develop a sense of coolness is very simple:

I know what I have to offer. Therefore, I know she is lucky to have me.

Let me explain. As an actress, I had to overcome a paralyzing fear of auditioning. When I first began to try out for movie roles, I was so nervous. I hated it. I went into the casting sessions desperate to figure out what the producers wanted me to be to be like in order to fit the role. I wanted them to like me and I was looking to them for approval of my worthiness. I was so terrified of being judged that I was doing the wrong thing or acting the wrong way or looking all wrong for the role that I would freeze up, tremble through my lines, and sometimes even break out into a flop sweat. When I didn't get the part—I mean, really, who would give someone a job who had a panic attack in the middle of the audition—I was totally devastated. It wasn't until I changed my mind-set that I began to nail auditions and land roles.

One day, I don't know what sparked it, probably something silly on *Dr. Phil*, but a lightbulb switched on in my brain, and I recalled what my dad told me on my first day of school. "Remember, kid, they're lucky to have you." I suddenly realized I was approaching the audition process ass backward. I was pushing. I was working too hard. I was self-conscious and overthinking. I was going into casting offices desperate instead of confident. I was needy to be liked instead of knowing why I was likeable. I began making a list of reasons why the casting directors were "lucky to have me" before my auditions. Everything changed. The new cool and confident me would walk into the casting office knowing I had something good to offer the production. I had a certain skill, or a style, or a life experience that could bring the role to life. I had a point of view and my "take" on the character instead of what I thought they thought I should be like. Also, in the process of making the list, I realized that the casting director was not the enemy. They need the role cast. It's their job. They're hoping I'm great so they can call it a day and go have happy hour with their friends. They're not the big bad judges I had made them out to be. They were not staring at me and picking apart all my faults. They were actually on my side. Auditioning became fun instead of terrifying. If I got the part, great! If not, it was not meant to be and I'd move on to the next one. It wasn't personal. It wasn't life or death. It wasn't a desperate situation. It just was. I became cool with it.

The same is true for meeting women. A date is just like an audition. You need to know your strengths and what you have to offer so you are grounded, cool, and collected when you come face-to-face with your leading lady. When you are confident, you don't have to try so hard. Understand that the Hot Chick you're trying to get into the sack is not the enemy. She's on your side. She doesn't notice all your little imperfections you're obsessing about. She is hoping you're a great guy so she has a date for next Saturday night and the one after that and the one after that so she can stop auditioning potential boyfriends and just be with you already!

Get out that notebook. You already made a list of the one hundred characteristics your Dream Girl has. Now, I want you to write down twenty reasons why this imaginary perfect girl is *lucky to have you*. It may seem stupid. Do it anyway. Don't think—just write. Twenty really isn't that big of a number. Remember, you came up with one hundred for her. I know, it may be difficult to praise yourself. If you can't come up with any reasons your Dream Girl would be lucky to have you, here are a few examples to get you started:

I love women.

I am fun to be around.

I make a great omelet.

I give good foot rubs.

I play a mean Rock Band.

I can bench press 120.

I'm creative.

I'm kind.

I'm a great joke teller.

I am a champion thumb wrestler.

I love to laugh.

I cry at sad movies.

I can BBQ with the best of them.

I can pay my bills.

I know all the words to "Tangled Up In Blue."

I do a great Christopher Walken impression.

I am able and willing to write a list of my good qualities.

I smell good.

I eat healthfully.

I dress well!

If you can think of more than twenty, great! Write them down. Yes. It's OK if they are silly reasons. Yes. You must write them down. I'm waiting.

* * *

Rah! Rah! Sis boom bah! I'm doing my jump splits for you in my little cheerleading outfit for a job well done.

Who knew you had so many great qualities? Now that you've acknowledged them, they have become real. They're out there. Own them. They make you the unique, lovable, attractive man that you are.

OK. I trust you have been doing your mantra from section one: *"I'm a great guy. I deserve a great woman."* Good. Now add in some of your specifics from your "Why She's Lucky to Have Me" list. *"I'm a great guy because I write good love poems. I deserve a hot woman because I will treat her with respect."* Add your specific qualities into your reprogramming. Every morning, while you're shaving, I want you to stand in front of the mirror, look yourself in the eye, and say why your Dream Girl is lucky to have you:

"She's lucky to have me because I treat her like a princess."

"She's lucky to have me because I am honest."

"She's lucky to have me because I love to eat pussy!"

Say it like you mean it, until you actually do.

I know. It seems dorky. The reprogramming process in itself isn't the hippest thing in the world. But trust me, it will ultimately help you get your cool on. When it sinks in and you finally start to realize what a great guy you are, so will the girl of your dreams. You'll begin to walk into rooms with an air of strength about you. You'll be at ease. You'll be "in the zone." You won't care what everyone else is thinking. You won't be worried about impressing anyone because you know who you are and what you have to offer, so they are, of course, lucky to have you. When you're truly confident, unlike Albert Brooks' character in *Broadcast News,* you'll never let them see you sweat. When you're cool, the hot women will be magnetically drawn to you.

Remember, there are no sure bets in life. Sometimes we will not be noticed, not be liked, or not get chosen. We have to conquer the fear of this rejection because the reality of it won't go away. It's how we handle ourselves in the face of this fear—how we fall down and learn to get back up—that makes us who we are. If one girl doesn't think you're cool that does not define your coolness. It's being able to move on to another woman that will, with what you've learned, that is the true test of confidence.

BIG P.S.

There are no shortcuts to confidence. There are no tricks you can play. There are no rules to feign cool. We hot women know *the game*. We can tell if you've been reading those pick–up books for guys. We've read them! *Your game is lame*. It's offensive. You cannot win if you try to *play* us. We're smarter than that. So keep reading to learn how to score from a woman's perspective.

Bottom Line: There's a girl out there who will be lucky to have a great guy like you!

TIME OUT

The first part of this book is mostly about preparing yourself to go out and win your girl. I've given you a lot of knowledge that you must not only understand but also put into action. You most likely have some homework to do. A trip to the drug store and men's department is probably in order. You may need to join the gym, start eating better, or clean up your house. You cannot just think about doing these things. You must actually *do* them. Before moving on, I want you to review these first three chapters and make a list of anything you need to change about yourself to help attract your perfect girl…and then start doing them if you haven't done so already. I also want you to reread your list of your perfect mate's traits and ask yourself this question: Are you a guy that your Dream Girl would go out with? Or, do you need to make some improvements? Remember, needing to fix something is not a negative. It's a positive. Taking specific actions that make you more "dateable" is a necessary step toward getting what you want. Now, put the book down and get done what needs to be done so you are ready to *go get her!*

Step 4: GO GET HER

I go where she goes. – Grandpa

When I asked my grandfather the secret to how he met my grandmother, he said, *"That's easy. I go where she goes."* When he saw my pretty little grandma-to-be on his first day of high school, my grandpa-to-be wasted no time. He immediately enrolled in all her classes, including home economics, in which he was the only boy and had absolutely no interest in— except for the girl. He joined the choir because she sang in it. He ran for student council because she was secretary. His plan seems to have worked as they got married, had babies, and lived happily ever after for over sixty-five years.

Chances are you understand that you're not going to find your Dream Girl while sitting on the couch, eating Doritos, and surfing the net for porn. If you want to find your perfect woman, you must leave the house and make yourself available. *Don't* go to the sports bar because there are too many dudes. *Don't* visit the titty bars because "Desiree" is only saying you're cute because you're paying for lap dances and her bottomless Jack and Diet Cokes. What you do need to do is go to where the available girls are.

You may know who you're after. If so, be like Grandpa and simply go where she goes. Don't get me wrong. I'm not encouraging you to be a stalker. But if you notice the Hot Chick from the PR department likes to make Starbucks runs at eleven a.m., maybe you should pick up a latte habit. If you don't have a girl in mind, you need to find one and then stalk her—just kidding. No, seriously. Don't be a psycho freak.

Here are my favorite places for meeting the ladies:

Dance, Pilates, or Yoga Classes

Group fitness classes are great for meeting women. You'll not only work muscles you didn't even know you had, but you'll also be in heaven for an hour in the midst of hot, barely-dressed, sweat-glistening girls. If you've never been to a workout class, don't be afraid of looking silly. The ladies will think you're brave for trying something new. Just don't overdo it and hurt yourself. Let's face it, where else can you go where men are outnumbered by lean, strong, flexible women ten to one. If you're hitting the gym classes to meet girls, be sure to go after work hours. Lunchtime classes are for housewives. Nighttime is the right time for meeting available women. Also, any dance class that requires a partner, like swing or tango, is a sure bet. Just show up and they'll match you with another single. Just don't get stuck with the seventy-year-old, 200-pound grandma. Be sure to beeline to the cute wallflower flying solo and tell her that "Nobody puts Baby in a corner." You'll be her instant dreamboat. Even if you don't meet your Cinderella at the ballroom class, you'll learn a great skill for future weddings, parties, etc. Which brings us to…

Weddings, Parties, etc.

Don't worry if you're invited to a wedding and you don't have a date. Weddings are a great place to meet girls. Everyone's celebrating love, drinking, and dancing the night away. They're a fantastic breeding ground for romance—or, at least a drunken fling in the coat check room. Weddings and other parties are wonderful because you already have something in common with all the female guests—you have a mutual friend who invited you. "So, how do you know the host (or the bride or groom)" is a perfect conversation starter. It's totally OK to arrive at any party alone.

I know it's hard sometimes to make a solo entrance, but remember, no one is staring at you and judging you for being by yourself. They're all too busy worrying about what you are thinking about them.

This is what is going through a woman's brain when you walk into a party:

"How's my hair?"

"Do I look fat in this dress?"

"Will anyone ask me to dance?"

"Did I feed the cat?"

"Where's the guy with the little shrimp ball thingies?"

(You enter)

"Oooh! Is he single?"

"He's kinda cute."

"Oh my God. I do I look fat in this dress. I shouldn't have had so many shrimp thingies. Diet starts now... Well, after the leftover birthday cake is gone."

"Is he looking at me?"

"I hope he comes over and says hello."

Beautiful, single women love to see an unattached guy like you walk into the room because YOU are what they are ALL after: *a put together, available man.* Just remember, you're a great catch. You're clean, you dress well, you're healthy, and she's lucky to have you. You're like filet mignon to a pack of hungry dogs. You'll have to fight those bitches off!

Language or Cooking Classes

It's true: women are turned on by men who wear aprons and can make more than toast and ramen noodles. These types of interactive classes throw you in a room full of women who have come together in the name of self-improvement. It's an ideal place to meet a woman who is obviously single because she has time for such activities.

Not only do you get to meet women and spend time with them, these classes also give you a perfect excuse to ask her over to your place to practice your new recipes or quiz each other on Spanish vocabulary words. Find classes in your area online. Some savvy places may even offer singles nights. Even if you don't meet your perfect girl in class, you can learn the skills to impress future babes with your mastery of homemade pesto or your ability to roll a Romance language off your tongue.

The Grocery Store Health Aisle

Everyone says the grocery store is a great place to meet women. But you can't just push your cart around hoping to run into your future wife. You need a plan, so I'm going to give you one. You need at least an hour. You need to go to Whole Foods or the closest health-related market nearest you; go to the vitamin aisle and look at the food supplements. I'm talking vitamins, herbs, and essential fatty acids. All that stuff gives you a reason to hang out to study ingredients… and scope for Hot Chicks. This is where the women that care about their bodies go. This is the Hot Chick section the supermarket. Do not hang around browsing the digestive dysfunction remedies because it is *so* not sexy. Look at something general, like a B-complex or time-release Vitamin C capsule. Read the labels until a really hot, fit woman comes along. Then, ask her if she's tried it and what she thinks. It may seem horrifying to actually look a sexy, in-shape woman in her eyes and speak. However, it is a legitimate conversation starter. What to do next will be discussed in future chapters.

Art Galleries and Museums

It's a no-brainer. At an art gallery or museum you already have something to talk about: the art piece in front of you. Who cares if you're not into French impressionism and you don't know why a can of Campbell's soup could be worth a zillion dollars. If Hot Chicks dig looking at overpriced wall decorations, then so should you. Have fun with it. Let your inner left bank artiste out to play. Just be sure to do a little research on the exhibit you're planning to attend. You don't want to attribute *Starry Night* to Van *Halen*.

Eating Alone at a Restaurant

Eating at the bar at an upscale restaurant is a great way to meet women. Just show up in your hot-guy sport coat uniform and situate yourself next to the pretty single lady eating alone. If she has a magazine and turns her back to you, she's not interested. If you're in a hotel bar and she's wearing a mini skirt and lets you know she isn't wearing any panties, she's probably a hooker. If she's looking around, making eye contact with you, and actually consuming food, not just martini olives, she is hoping you'll buy her a drink, talk to her, and ask her out. No, really. She's there because she wants to meet the man of her dreams. That man could be you.

Building Supply and Hardware Stores

Many women, including me, don't know the difference between a nut and a bolt let alone a Makita or a monkey wrench. If you want to find a girl to nail, it may be of use to talk caulk. Most women wander around hardware stores with very little idea of what they are doing. If she looks like she's trying to figure out which contraption to buy, it's totally fine to approach her and offer a suggestion. If she seems open to it, ask her if she needs help with anything else. Ask her what she is trying to build or fix? Then guide her to anything else she may need. It's the perfect opportunity to show off your manliness and rescue a damsel in distress. You can also give her your number and offer your handyman services just in case she has any trouble nailing her rack to the wall or snaking her drain.

The Dog Park

Have a dog? Great! Go to the dog-park or hiking canyon where all the hot chicks walk their pups, and use your cute canine to attract the lassies that also love four-legged friends. But remember, a sophisticated woman will not drool over your puppy-mill pug or untrained, bully bulldog. If you get a dog, it should be a rescue animal and preferably a well-mannered creature that is not bigger than she is. You will win a woman's heart with the heroic story of how you saved your sweet-ole-boy from a high kill shelter, or purchased your fluffy new puppy from humane rescue pet store like Shelter Hope Pet Shop. ShelterHopePetShop. org.

Shopping in a Department Store

Warning: Do not try this unless you are very charming. This approach takes a lot of balls. Pretend you're shopping for your sister or some other imaginary non-threatening woman, like your executive assistant or something. Ask an attractive female shopper, who is browsing near you, for her opinion on what you should buy as a gift. Give her a choice, like: *"If this were a present for you, would you go for the sweater or the blouse?"* Don't be shopping in the lingerie section. She'll immediately peg you as a creep-a-zoid. Go basic, like the accessories section. *"What do you think would make a better gift? The tote bag or the clutch?"* Most women enjoy giving advice. She will get the idea that you are a caring guy who likes to buy thoughtful gifts for the ladies in your life. Don't push your luck by asking her to try it on or model it for you unless you really get an open vibe and you are one hundred percent willing to buy one for her if she likes it.

Yoga Retreat or Away-From-Home Workshop

We already know yoga classes are great places to meet hot women. You can take it up a notch by making it a sleepover. Yoga retreats and other self-help spiritual or health seminars are packed with single women looking to find meaning in their lives. When women are away from the constraints of social norms, like a seaside or south-of-the-border eco-retreat with you being the only single guy in the vicinity who speaks English, anything can happen. After a full day of downward dogs, scantily clad dips in the ocean, and sunset meditation walks along *la playa*, the nights will give way to bonfire fiestas and tequila tasting. You may think energy aligning with crystals is a bunch of hooey; however, if you can help unclog a women's root chakra beneath a mosquito net in Mexico, it may be worth the trip.

Online

I know there's still a lingering stigma to online dating. But, I've done it with success. I'm not saying get your credit card out and join a generic dating website. There are too many weeds to sort through, and those sites that pair you according to some dumb quiz you take are pretty useless if you ask me. When it comes to matters of the heart, there are no standardized tests. I also don't recommend spending thousands of dollars on an overpriced "matchmaker" that is just going to throw a bunch of girls at you and hope that one sticks. Instead, know the kind of girl you want and go on a website that caters to that woman. Get out your list. I'm waiting, so go get it…

* * *

You know what you want because you've written it down. If you know what kind of girl you want, there is a website out there to find her. Search *dating + something on your list.*

For example: If a woman who *"loves to be spoiled"* is one of the qualities of your perfect girl, try typing *"dating + loves to be spoiled."* You will probably be directed to someplace like MillionaireMatch.com.

Need a nice Jewish girl to take home to Mom? Then search *"dating + Jewish"* and you'll probably end up at some semblance of JDate.com.

Have kids and want someone who does too? Try *"women dating + single parent"* and you'll probably land on the Parents Without Partners parentswithoutpartners.org home page.

Like to be tied up and spanked or tying up and doing the spanking? Then, type in *"dating + BDSM"* and you'll be smack dab at the home page of alt.com an alternative lifestyles dating site.

Get as specific as you can. *"Dating +Spoiled + Jewish + Single Parent + BDSM"* probably leads to a site to meet just that kind of girl. God bless the Internet!

Even if you think online dating is not for you, I urge you to do a little browsing anyway. Seeing for yourself how many women are out there looking for a mate is encouraging. Who knows, you might just come across a profile of that former co-worker that you had a crush on that you never asked out or reconnect with the one-who-got-away high school sweetheart who is now divorced and available for you. Then all you have to do is:

Ask her out!

Mike: *"I don't know you very well, you know, but I wanted to ask you—how'd you get Diane Court to go out with you?"*

Lloyd: *"I called her up."*

Mike: *"But how come it worked? I mean, like, what are you?"*

Lloyd: *"I'm Lloyd Dobler."*

Mike: *"This is great. This gives me hope. Thanks."*

–Say Anything

I love the early Cameron Crowe teen-romance flick *Say Anything*. It's a sweet story of noble underachiever (John Cusack as Lloyd Dobler) and a beautiful valedictorian (Ione Skye as Diane Court) falling in love the summer before she goes off to college. It's a great example of a not-so-hot guy getting a super-hot girl to go out with him. How? *He asked.* He knew who he was and who he wanted. Then he simply went after her—with gusto. Now, so must you. If you haven't seen the movie, get it. Watch it. Learn from Lloyd.

You're already well on your way to making the bold move of asking a hot woman out on a date You've learned a lot, starting with knowing that it's possible. You also know what kind of girl you want and what you have to offer her. You've also made the effort to package yourself to attract a great woman. You even know where to go to find the woman of your dreams. Now, all you need to do is muster the guts to ask her out. I encourage you to continue with your affirmations through this crucial stage of putting the knowledge you've acquired into the action. It's a good idea to change your mantra so it's fresh, and gear it toward the actual act of asking a girl out on a date like this:

"Hot women love to go out with me because… (Something from your why-they're-lucky-to-have-you list)"

"Hot women give me their number because…I'm funny."

"Hot women say yes to a date with me because…I'm generous. "

"Hot women are attracted to me because…I'm respectful."

This is also a good time to add to the list of things you have to offer. I bet you can add another ten reasons why a sexy woman would want to go on a date with you. After all, you're following the tried and true steps that this hot woman is sharing with you. If you've been diligent thus far, I have a good feeling you will be successful. And, I'm rooting for you!

I have a simple *Ask Her Out Formula* to get your Dream Girl to say "yes" to a date with you.

Here is what you do:

Make Eye Contact

Smile

Say Hello

Give Her a Compliment

Ask a Question

Ask Her Out

REALLY. IT'S THAT SIMPLE. It's not brain surgery. It's not magic. It's easy. Let me break it down for you.

Make Eye Contact

Eye contact is essential if you want to connect with a woman. It's a powerful communication that says loud and clear "I like what I see." It tells her she has caught your eye. Eye contact does not mean stare her down like a hungry tiger eying his prey. Looking a woman in the eyes is very intimate and at the same time aggressive. It also compels her to look back at you. Eye contact is where it all begins. Let it linger for the count of three. One one thousand…Two one thousand…three one thousand…and then…

Smile

Smiling is contagious. It works wonders. So many people go around not smiling that when you do smile you'll stick out like a neon pink T-shirt at a funeral. If you smile, you will shine and she will notice. She'll think, *"Wow. What a nice guy. I wish I knew him,"* and she'll smile back. If she holds eye contact and smiles, you're in. She's interested. Game on. That's your cue to approach her and...

Say Hello

Really it's OK. People can talk to each other. Believe me, you won't be struck by lightning for saying hello to a pretty girl. I know it may seem daunting to be so bold as to speak to a real live beautiful woman. The best way to avoid a panic attack when doing so is to practice. Go for a walk. Don't look down and frown like everyone else in town. Instead, do the opposite. Engage with the women around you. Say "Hi" to the lovely lady instead of hoping she doesn't notice your unshaven face and dirty T-shirt. You're beyond that. You're the new you. You're wearing your clean, crisp, casual uniform and know that you have something to offer. So, be like Lloyd. Say hello. *Say anything.*

Give Her a Compliment

It's basic human psychology. If you make a woman feel good about herself, she will in turn feel good about you. A woman may fain not to care when you tell her you "love the freckles on her shoulders." But, take it from someone who knows, she will remember every word you say if it is a genuine observation. Unique compliments about qualities that are important to her self-esteem will indeed *get you everywhere,* especially when the woman is über-sexy.

For example: That statuesque, buxom Brazilian may respond well when you compliment her looks. But, believe me, she'll cream when you compliment her intelligence, her voice, her smile, or whatever you sense is an important quality that most people will overlook because she is so smokin' hot. Just don't go overboard and compare her to the *Mona Lisa* or quote Shakespeare or any other ridiculous over-the-top lameness. Women will easily detect if a compliment is your standard pickup line. Don't bother. That kind of fake flattery will *get you nowhere.*

Ask a Question

Asking questions keeps conversation going. Don't ask yes and no questions about meaningless things like, *"So, do you come here often?"* or *"Nice weather we're having, eh?"* Ask real questions that show you are interested in her—for more than her great rack—like *"I noticed your iPad. I was thinking of getting one. What do you like about it?"* or *"I see you ride your bike to work. That's cool. How'd you get into that?"* Questions based on actual observations about your lady of interest will put her at ease and show her you genuinely have noticed her and like her for who she is.

This is the secret special trick, guys, so pay attention. Compliments are nice, but they are especially potent when paired with a question. Why? Because it initiates conversation. If you give a compliment-wrapped question to a woman, it prompts her to answer. You can then engage her in a chat with further questions about something that genuinely pertains to her and that she's interested in sharing. Don't talk about something random like the weather. Instead, talk about her. It will actually lead to something. Here is an example of a compliment-question hybrid:

You say: I noticed your arms. They're really toned. Do you do yoga?

She says: Oh. Thanks. Uh… yes. I do.

You say: I just started going to classes. What kind do you do?

She says: Hatha Flow

You say: I heard of that. What is it exactly?

She says: It's a lot of linking postures and moving through poses. It's really fun, and a great workout.

You say: That sounds great. I could use a class like that. Where's a good place to go?

She says: Well, I like Rachel's class at Equinox.

You say: Cool. Do you know which days she teaches?

She says: She has a class Saturday afternoon.

You say: Oh, great, thanks. Are you going this Saturday?

She says: Uh… Maybe.

You say: Well. I hope to see you there sometime.

Congratulations! You just turned a cliché come-on line like *"You must work out"* into a potential go-where-she-goes-place, which can lead to an actual real live day-date.

Ask Her Out

Whether you meet her and connect right away or go where she goes to and establish a further connection, don't dillydally. Once you've engaged her in some serious one-on-one conversation—and I don't mean a drawn-out courtship of becoming friends, I just mean a few minutes alone where she is actually looking at you, smiling, and talking to you because you've followed the *Make Eye Contact-Smile-Say Hello-Give Her a Compliment-Ask a Question formula*—just do it. Get right to the point. Be direct and clear and positive. Don't be wishy-washy:

"I don't know. But, maybe, I mean, if you're not busy…we could hang out some time" will not get the job done. Be a man and state your business. I suggest using "I" messages when asking a woman out. For example:

"I really think you're great. I'd love to take you to dinner."

"I'm single. If you're available, I'd like to take you out sometime."

"I'd really like to take you out on a date. Could I please get your number so I can call you?"

It's not that hard. The worst that can happen is that she'll say:

"Thanks, but no thanks".

"Sorry, I have a boyfriend."

or

"I'm not interested."

Big deal. At least you know. At least you won't waste your time wondering what she'd say *if* you got up the nerve to ask her.

If she seems to make a lame blow-off excuse like, *"I'm really busy"* just be charmingly straightforward, smile, and say:

"Should I keep asking?"

If she's really not interested she'll say, *"Look, I'm not interested."*

However, you may have a shot if she says, *"Maybe another time."*

Just don't let the cat-and-mouse game drag on for more than a few weeks, or she's just having a hard time letting you down and you don't want to waste any more of your valuable time that could be spent in the arms of your Dream Girl.

Remember, one of the essential qualities that your perfect woman should have is that *She* is into *You*. If she's obviously not interested in you, then move on. There are plenty of other hot babes out there who would be lucky to have you. If *"She is totally into me"* or *"She likes me back"* or *"She is crazy about me"* is not on your list of qualities your Dream Girl possesses, get out your pen and paper and put them on the list now. Do it!

Signs She is Interested

I always get the question: *How do I know if she wants me to approach her?*

It's really not hard. Signs a woman is interested in you include the following:

She Wants You

She holds your eye contact—good sign she is available.

She smiles back—great sign she's interested in you.

She tilts her chin down, looks up with her eyes all girly, smiles…and blushes—sure thing she thinks you're hot too.

She Wants You to Leave Her Alone

If she *avoids* your eye contact—she's *not interested.*

If she *doesn't smile* back—she's *not interested.*

If she rolls her eyes, turns her back, shakes her head no, or moves to get away from you—*she's not interested*!

I'm gonna break it to you, buddy: *If you're not sure she's interested, she probably isn't.*

P.S. YES! It is your job as a man to pursue and ask the woman out. Accept that you are the chaser not the chasee. In the world of dating really hot women, not bimbo club chicks, I offer no poser techniques to get girls to come to you. You can be master of the scene and socially dominant blah blah blah, but that, on its own, will not get a sophisticated lady to go out with you. You must initiate the contact and present the invitation. You must go after her. That is the way it works, no ifs ands, or buts.

It's really not that difficult. The real work begins when she says yes.

Bottom Line: Your Dream Girl can never say "yes" to a date with you unless you get yourself together and ask.

Step 5: BE A GREAT DATE

He who fails to plan, plans to fail – Proverb

She said yes. Holy *!?@ Now what?

This is the moment you've been waiting for, so you have to be prepared for it. If your reaction to her saying "yes" to your invitation to go out is *"Uh, OK, great. Cool. Let's hang out sometime"* – IT WILL NEVER HAPPEN. You must actually make a date with her that involves a specific plan of action. It's called a date because it's a specific date on the calendar like, Saturday, July 25th at 7:30 p.m. A date is not a vague, distant future occurrence at an unknown time. A date is not at that moment or later that same evening, either. "What are you doing later?" is not Dream Girl-worthy. A woman wants to feel like she's worth waiting for and you don't want to come off desperate. Plus, you need time to plan what a Hot Chick will think is *A Great Night Out*.

To seal the deal, you need to *agree on the date and get her phone number.*

This is how it's done:

You say: *"I'd love to take you to dinner sometime."*

Never invite a hot woman to coffee or a drink. Do you think she's gonna get dressed up and save a slot in her busy schedule just for a cappuccino? No. Coffee is not a real date and just a drink is noncommittal. It says you're not serious. Lunch is sort of lame too. It's too safe and boring. She lunches with her girlfriends. You don't want to be her friend; you want to be her lover. Dinner is serious business. So…

You say: *"I'd love to take you to dinner sometime."*

She says: *"That would be nice."*

You say: *"Great, how's this Saturday for you?"*

She says: *"Saturday's good."*

Or if

She says: *"I'm busy this weekend."*

You say: *"When is good for you?"*

There's nothing wrong with a Wednesday night dinner. Just get her to commit to a day. Then:

You say: *"Great, let me get your number so I can call you."*

You have to get her number. If she doesn't give you her number, move on because she's not interested, not available, or both. Giving her your card with your name, phone number, and e-mail on it is helpful. It will help her feel comfortable sharing her info with you because now she has yours. If you don't have a business card, go out and get one made. It's crucial to your success in getting dates with hot women.

Do not settle for *"I'll call you."*

It's a blow-off. If she really wants to go out with you, she'll give you her number. Not an e-mail address, not a Facebook profile, but seven digits that actually reach her directly. Once you have her number in hand or added to your iPhone, it's time to wrap it up and get out of there before you screw it up. Don't linger. She's a busy woman, and you've got places to go and people to see. If you don't, act like you do. Then…

You say: *"Thanks. Do you like Italian?*

I mean who doesn't like Italian? It's a safe bet she'll say yes. All chicks dig Italian food. It's romantic. That's where the word *romance* comes from: Rome. Unless she is some kind of raw food, vegan, hippie, health food nutcase (and then you don't really want to go out with her anyway because she probably doesn't groom down there), she'll love a table for two at your favorite ristorante. So…

She says: *"Yes. I love Italian."*

You say: *"I'll call you to confirm the time. Looking forward to it. Bye."*

The deal is officially sealed. See? That's not so hard.

Now we know that you're not out there collecting numbers just to collect numbers. You're going to plan a great dinner and then call her back to confirm the details. Of course, you can't just wing it and expect everything to go well. You need to make sure everything goes as smoothly as possible, so here are the basics.

Prep the Place

Never show up at random restaurant without a reservation. Duh! Picking a familiar place where you are known and liked is the best scenario for a first date. Call the hostess and ask for your favorite table on the date and at the time you want it. When you are familiar with the place, the hostess will greet you by name. When you are a regular, the owner or manager may stop by the table to say hello or send over a complimentary appetizer or dessert. These personal touches make you look like *The Man*—because you are. You're in with them. You're a good customer and, therefore, respected, which shows your date that you're a good guy.

When you're comfortable in the place, you will be comfortable in your own skin.

There is already a component of nerves from the newness of the situation—going on a first date with your hot woman of choice. Keep the rest under your control as much as possible. If you don't have a go-to favorite restaurant, find one, or several, in your area. Look up the "top ten date restaurants" in your city on your favorite search engine. Or, ask friends where they like to go to get a recommendation from someone you know. Go to the places on your own or with a friend. Eat there or at least get the lay of the land, feel the vibe, and taste something from their kitchen. Pick your favorites and then file them as great places to take dates. Know the best route to get to the place, where to park, where the restrooms are, and what's best on the menu and wine list. The more knowledgeable you are about the place, the better experience you can share with your sizzling hot date.

When picking the place, you are aiming for nice and intimate, not over-the-top fancy or loud and clubby. Romantic lighting, cozy atmosphere, and soft music are good. Stark lighting, hurried atmosphere, and loud music are bad. Don't over impress by planning a tasting menu and wine pairing extravaganza the first time out. You want to be able to wear your uniform, not a suit. She should be at home in jeans *or* a simple black dress.

Also, women get wary if they think you are trying too hard. Remember, desperation is not a turn-on. They also don't like to feel like you're trying to buy them just so they owe you something. Whether the wine is fifteen dollars or fifteen hundred dollars, she's not going to go home with you unless she really likes you. So, go easy, champ. Save some for the second round: date number two.

Prep Her

Call to solidify the details within a day of making the date. If her voice mail picks up, simply say:

"Hi It's X. I have a reservation for our date and want to give you the details. Please call me. My number is...310... blah blah blah."

It's better to confirm person-to-person rather than leave her a message. Too many things can go wrong like:

She gets the message of where and when but doesn't show up because she's waiting at her place for you to pick her up.

Or

She accidentally erases the message and doesn't have your number to call you back.

Or

She didn't get the message and thinks you've stood her up.

Or

She got the message but doesn't call you back and stands you up.

Meanwhile, you're sitting in the restaurant by yourself wondering where she is because you left a message with the details so you're assuming it's on. Be sure to talk to her, so you're both crystal clear. Once you have her on the phone, tell her the name of the restaurant and the time of the reservation. Offer to pick her up. If she says, *"Great. Pick me up,"* do it. Get her address and map it ahead of time so you know where you are going and how long you'll need to get there. Depending on where she lives, hopefully not an hour-and-a-half away in the opposite direction in traffic, decide on a time you will pick her up.

Ninety percent of the time on a first date your Dream Girl will want to meet you at the restaurant. Don't be offended and don't pressure her to ride with you. The reason a hot woman doesn't want some guy she barely knows coming to her house is that she is used to having people fall in love with her all the time and she doesn't need another whack-job showing up on her doorstep. She is assuming you are the worst-case scenario in order to protect herself. If it turns out you are indeed crazy, a pervert, or a scumbag, she doesn't want you to know where she lives. She feels safer meeting you there. If you do persist in getting her to ride with you, she will likely cancel because she thinks you are pushy and a stalker.

Chances are you're meeting her at the restaurant. Give her the address and offer a website, if there is one, so she can look into it herself. Also, if there are more than two days between the time you make the date and the date itself, follow up with a phone call the afternoon the day of. Leaving a message is fine:

"Hi. It's (Mike). Looking forward to seeing you tonight at 7:30. 310.555.4321."

It may sound silly, but it's good manners to confirm. You also give her your number again in case she's lost it and needs it for whatever reason. It also just plain reminds her it's all happening. A first date is awkward enough and no one wants to be a flake or flaked upon. Don't be needy and insecure:

"Hi. It's me. I'm just checking in to make sure we're still on for Saturday? Um, call me OK just so I know... either way. Uh, bye."

Don't do that! You're giving her a reason to cancel. If you're wishy-washy and whiney, she'll think you're a needy loser and bail out on the date. Also, it's a first date and she barely knows you so *"It's just me"* may not ring any bells. Be considerate and to-the-point. She'll probably give a call back or a quick text: *"Yes. See you there."* Just be direct and she'll think you're a nice, responsible, considerate person who she's looking forward to spending a nice evening with.

Prep Yourself

As soon as you make the date, your plan is put into action. You must make sure the place is right and your sexy girlfriend-to-be is well-prepped. However, don't forget to take care of you.

Do you need to cancel that ball game you said you would watch with your buddies? Or, do you need to reschedule that drink meeting to an hour earlier to give yourself time to get to the restaurant ten minutes early to make sure your table is ready? Do you need to pick up your favorite sport coat from the cleaners? Get a haircut? Gas up and wash your car? There's plenty to do before your big night, and you don't want to leave it to the last minute.

Practice Your Positive Spin

As the date night draws near, keep your composure by continuing your affirmations to remind yourself why she's lucky to have you. It never hurts to brush up on your conversation skills, especially if you haven't been on a date this millennium. You can even practice making small talk with the mirror. After all, do you have a response to *"So tell me about yourself?"*

Not that you want an overly rehearsed, pat answer, but it is helpful to practice a "Positive Pitch" of yourself. Create your pitch from your good qualities list and newly improved lifestyle you've implemented from reading this book. Give her a taste of the general good things about you that won't cause controversy and will encourage her to like you. For example:

She says: *"So, tell me about yourself."*

You say: *"I enjoy good food."*

"I like to travel."

"I love going to concerts."

You know, the sweet, basic, noncontroversial stuff.

If you aren't happy with your life at the moment—because you've just moved out of your parents' basement and finally got a job after being laid off for a year-and-a-half and after having already lost your house in a horrible divorce—for God's sake, don't tell her! Don't explain what a terrifying shambles your life had become and how you're really not as pathetic as your ex-wife says you are. Instead, tell her that you are excited about a new chapter in your life. You have a budding career and you're leasing a great little apartment until you find the perfect woman to settle down and go house-hunting with. Practice the positive spin so you're able to present yourself to your Dream Girl in the best possible light.

Believe it or not, you have everything you need to be a great first date because you have followed my steps so far. In order to keep her interested and avoid having a drink thrown in your face, I'm giving you some *First Date Tips and Rules*.

Be Interested In More Than Her Breasts

Yes. She has great rack and you can't wait to get your hands on them. However, take it from a woman who has both big breasts and brains, we are immediately turned off if we have to say,

"Hey, buddy, my eyes are up here."

We want to know that you are into us for more than our body and that you are more evolved than a Neanderthal.

No Looking Around At Other Women

It's the first date, for crying out loud. All your focus should be on the girl you are with. OK, if that Victoria's Secret model you've been whacking off to just happens to walk by, you have a free pass—I'd probably drop my jaw too. But seriously, checking out other Hot Chicks when you're with one is a big no-no. A wandering eye is a loud and clear alarm that you are a player and/or a cheater so we'll want nothing to do with you.

Avoid Phone Calls

Men addicted to their Crackberries are not hot. We don't think you're more of a bigwig because you get a continual stream of "very important" phone calls. We actually think you're less impressive because you don't have a full-time, highly trained, dedicated staff to answer your phone and take care of business for you. We hot women don't want to hear *"It's an emergency. I have to take this"* unless it's life or death. A life-or-death example is the following:

> You're an OB/GYN and your patient is going into labor any minute, and the complications of

the breeched baby could kill them both if you don't answer the phone and talk them through it immediately.

If this sort of actual emergency is the case, you must explain to your date beforehand that you may be getting a life-or-death matter phone call and tell her what it is regarding. If it is not literally a life-or-death emergency situation, *let it go to voice mail.* If you are expecting an important business e-mail or call from someone you've been trying to get a hold of all week and they finally call you back in the middle of dinner, *let it go to voice mail.* If you must, check your PDA messages in the bathroom later. But if you're gone longer than five minutes, don't be surprised if your date disappears. Remember, the only thing that is important right now is the woman in front of you. You will never make it to the second date if you don't pay attention on the first.

Mind Your Manners

I don't want to sound like your kindergarten teacher, but mind your Ps and Qs and chew with your mouth closed. A great way to turn off a lady is to eat like a beast and belch like an ogre. Also, you may think it old-fashioned, but as a rule it's "Ladies First." She walks ahead of you, sits before you, and orders before you. Some guys think modern women don't care if you open their door, stand when they stand, or say "Bless you" when they sneeze— they're wrong. Women want you to be chivalrous and charming. Your date is not your buddy to hang out with. She is your special guest and should be treated as such.

FYI: These rules apply to every date. Not just the first. Yes, the rules apply to you too.

Five Easy Conversations for a Great First Date

Let's assume you follow the rules so your hot date doesn't ditch you while you've stepped away to make another "important" phone call. However, now you have to actually keep the conversation going past drinks and an appetizer selection.

Simply talking can sometimes be trying on a first date because you don't really know each other and don't have shared experiences to relate. There are some common traps you can fall into, like the huge gap of silence that feels like an eternity even though it is really only seven seconds. Here are suggestions for small talk beyond the typical *"So, tell me about yourself."*

Talk About Her

Remember the question-and-compliment formula from Step 4? Good. Just as it's a great way to launch a first chat, it's perfect for keeping the conversation sailing smoothly. If lost for words, you can always give her a sincere compliment. Notice her style and presentation and make it a talking point. Like this:

"I love your dress. Who makes it?"

"I noticed your handbag. Is that a designer you like?"

"You smell great. What's the perfume you're wearing?"

Listen and take mental notes. Not only is it good small talk, the information she gives you is useful for planning future gifts like:

A scarf by the designer that makes her dress

A wallet that matches her bag

A bottle of her favorite fragrance

Not only will you be assured she will like the presents, but she'll feel like you're perceptive, knowing, and thoughtful. All these are qualities that help to make her want to throw you down on the bed.

Talk About the Place

Believe it or not, a great conversation can come about by simply talking about what's around you. You can talk about how you discovered the restaurant, how you know the chef that came by to say *"Buona Serra,"* a funny story about the waiter, yada yada yada. Tell her how much you love Italian food and why. Tell her how the olive oil there is almost as good as in Italy at this little bottega you once visited outside of Sienna, blah blah blah. Ask her if she's ever been to Italy. If she has, ask her where? If not, tell her about your favorites. Just don't make up tall tales. You don't want to be caught in a lie. If you've never been to Italy, tell her that ever since you saw that movie *Under the Tuscan Sun*, you can't wait to go to experience it for yourself. (Yes, if you haven't seen it, do. It's a chick flick, but a great first date Italian restaurant conversation.)

Notice your surroundings. What's around you can be a good conversation starter.

You say: *"I love that painting. The colors are so rich. Do you like art?"*

She says: *"Yes"* and then goes on a rant about how much she loved seeing the Botticelli's at the Uffizi in Florence.

And so it goes. If you use what's around you, the hot babe in front of you, the food, the decor, the wine, whatever, it will most likely inspire a more in-depth conversation that helps you get to know each other.

Talk About You

Give her the "I'm a great guy" version of the real you. Let her know what fun things you like to do. Tell her:

About the Monday night wine tasting you go to regularly.

That you like to go biking on the beach path.

How much you like going to movies the old-fashioned way—to the theatre.

Maybe she'll says she loves wine tastings, wishes she dusted off the Rollerblades and went to the beach more often, and thinks movies in the theatre are always better than on DVD too. Boom! You just created three great date possibilities by sharing what a fun guy you are—aka why she's lucky to have you. Also, if there is anything important about your life she should know, now's the time to bring it up. If you have a five-year-old son who lives with you, she should know that up front. You don't want to give your first date hottie a calendar chart of which nights you won't be available this month due to your son's soccer games. However, if you mention you have a child, and she goes on to tell you any of the following, then, believe me, it's better to stop the train-wreck in its tracks:

> She gets "all weird" around kids,
>
> Her sister's "brats" are so annoying, or
>
> Her last boyfriend's "devil-child" sabotaged their relationship.

On the other hand, you may breathe easier when she tells you she loves kids, has one of her own, or at least doesn't bolt for the door after learning about yours.

When you share your important life information, she will, most likely, let you know about hers. When you share something substantial, it gives her permission to do the same. Beware: she may reveal something about herself that is a deal breaker, like *"My stalker ex-boyfriend just got out of jail, so if you see a six foot four, 240-pound dude with a dragon tattooed on his neck, look out."* Again, better to know now.

Talk About Common Interests

If you met at a place of mutual interest like an "I Go Where She Goes" place, you always have that to chat about like:

"Have you been practicing your Spanish?"

"So what's your favorite recipe from cooking class?"

"What did you think of spinning Thursday?"

It makes for good small talk and can perhaps lead to a future trip to

> a Mexican restaurant,

> a date to practice your recipes, or

> a meet-up at the next workout class.

Then, there's the one thing that everyone has in common: *music*. Have you ever met anyone who doesn't like music? When all else fails, talk to her about what kind of music she likes. Ask:

"What are you favorite bands?"

"What have you downloaded lately from iTunes?"

or

"Do you like going to see live music? ... Rock concerts? ... Classical concertos? ...Jazz clubs?"

People tend to be passionate about their music, and if you find a common bond there, she'll feel like you're super cool, that you really "get" her, and that you may be the guy she's been dying to meet. It's easy. For example:

You say: What are some of your all-time favorite bands?

She says: I love Counting Crows.

You say: Oh yeah, me too.

She says: *August and Everything After* is on my top ten albums ever.

You say: Yeah. That "Anna Begins" song gets me every time.

She says: Oh my God... I love that song. (Subtext: This guy is so cool. He likes Counting Crows so he understands *me*. He may be my perfect guy.)

You're in! You have formed a deep emotional bond just by appreciating the same music. It's a no-brainer.

Yes. If you don't own Counting Crows' *August and Everything After* download it, buy the CD, what have you—just get it! Listen and learn. Chicks love that shit. Just look at all the smokin' hot Hollywood babes who went out with Adam Duritz—and he's no looker.

Note what she enjoys musically for a future date or gift.

Talk More About Her

You want to find out what this girl is really all about? So, ask her questions that will determine if she is the kind of girl for you. What on your list of one hundred qualities your Dream Girl possesses does this girl possibly have? You don't want to go at her like the Spanish Inquisition and ask her how many kids she wants. You don't want to plan the wedding yet or you'll scare her off. However, you do want to find out if you have anything in common.

Don't ask for a life history. Don't ask about past relationships, old boyfriends, or ex-husbands. Her past life is *her* past life and it should stay there—in the past. It's none of your business unless she brings it up and wants to talk about it. It will only make you crazy, even if you say it won't. She doesn't want to hear about your ex-whatever either. Do ask her:

"What do you like to do on a typical night?"

"What activities or hobbies do you enjoy?"

"Where do you like to go away for the weekend?"

If her answers are along the lines of *"I love going out every night to the hot new clubs and trendy restaurants"* and your Dream Girl is someone who "loves staying in" and "enjoys old movies," you may not get very far. It's better to know now. Remember, you're not just trying to impress her. You're looking to see if she is someone *you* want to go out with more than once.

Avoid Probing

Did you get the part where I said *avoid talking about past relationships?* I'm just checking. It's fine to ask a general question about friends or family if it's genuine, like *"Do you have family in town?"* or *"Tell me about your friends."*

But don't attempt to psychoanalyze her. It's such a freshman move to try to "figure her out" from asking what her father was like. It's not about how to use whatever information she gives you to help get her into bed. It's about finding out if she is someone *you want* to take to bed. With the genuine approach, getting her in the sack is more likely anyway.

Also, even if you did Google her and found out X, Y, and Z...don't bring it up until dates two, three and four. Try to get to know her the good old-fashioned way first.

Another Word on EX-Wives, EX-Girlfriends, etc.

Did I mention DO NOT talk about an ex-girlfriend or past relationship if at all possible on a first date? If she asks, and only if she asks, then only say GOOD THINGS about your past lovers. Non-damaging, vague, unthreatening things like:

"It didn't work out."

"She was a great lady, but not for me."

or

"She wasn't the one."

Are all fine and dandy.

Never say she was:

"A slutty slut slut!"

"Mentally ill."

or

"A total nightmare."

…and then give the gory details.

Everyone has a past and we all get it that both parties have had past relationships. However, you never want to share too much information—especially if it's negative. A woman will NOT want to go out with a man who talks bad about an ex. She will be afraid he will do the same to her. Also, women have a code amongst other women. She will side with her "sister" and think you are the asshole if you make a negative, sexist comment, like *"She was a PMSing pyscho bitch."*

Twelve Ways to Be the Man

Yes. It is your duty to pick up the check. She didn't come up to you and say, "Hey Mister, I'd love to take you to dinner."

It was the other way around. You're *The Man.* Own it. Hot Chicks expect you to not only pay the bill but also to be a gentleman in all of the following ways:

1. **Open the door** for her. That goes for car doors too if you're driving her.

2. If she's meeting you there, **stand up** when you see her.

3. **Make contact**. Give her a cheek kiss or light squeeze hello.

4. **Wait until she's seated** to sit. Let her pick where she wants to sit—usually facing out.

5. Ask if she would like wine with dinner. If so, ask if she prefers white or red and then get a wine list. If you're familiar with the selections, **order a bottle of wine** that you like. If you are not, ask a sommelier for suggestions. DO NOT order shots. Do not get drunk!

6. **Make suggestions** if you know the restaurant well. However, do not order for her. Of course let her pick whatever she wants off the menu.

7. **Offer dessert** as well. Sharing one dessert with two spoons is very intimate and a good sign she likes you.

8. **Don't complain** about the service or the bill. After all, you picked the place and you don't want to be a downer.

9. Be nice to the service people and **be a good tipper**. Yes, she notices. Yes, twenty percent is standard.

10. Be assertive. If you like her, **make another date before you leave** the restaurant. If you don't have a plan yet, try this:

> **You say**: *"I had fun. I'd like to see you again."*
>
> If **She says**: *"Me too. That would be nice."*
>
> **You say**: *"Great. I'll call you this week."*
>
> If you do have a plan or specific date in mind, pop the question. For example:
>
> **You say**: *"I have tickets to the basketball game next Sunday. I'd love to take you. Are you available?"*

If you don't seal the deal for a second date, don't stress. You can always follow up with a phone call for a great round two. More details on that to come. If she answers your call or calls you back after you leave a message, you're in. After an unreturned second call, know she's not interested and move on to ask out a new Dream Girl.

Regardless of whether she agrees to a second date, you need to:

11. Walk her to her car and **pay for her valet ticket**. If you picked her up, drive her home. Don't send her home in a cab, even if it is across town and way out of your way.

12. Make the move for a kiss. If she's into you, she won't turn away for a cheek peck. **Give her a gentle on-the-lips kiss**. No tongue. Jamming your tongue down her throat like a fumbling thirteen-year-old boy will not turn her on. Tongue kissing is not sexy unless fully reciprocated in the heat of passion. It is not for first dates or for public places. If you jam your tongue down her throat, she will call her best girlfriend immediately and MAKE FUN OF YOU!

P. S. Do not ask her to come back to your place or if you can come in. If things go any further on the first date, it has to be her idea. She'll let the kiss linger into more of a make-out session. She'll ask you in for a drink if she's into it. Otherwise, leave her wanting more. A Hot Chick is so used to having to fight off drooling men with "stiffies" at the end of the evening that you don't want to push her for sex. The less you push, the more she'll be willing and wanting you in the near future. Remember, she isn't a rent-a-date from the escort service you used to call up. She isn't the sad girl you hooked up with at the neighborhood bar who puked all over your shoes. She's a bona fide Babe-a-rella and you don't want to just *wham-bam-thank-you-ma'am* her. You want her to like you, go out with you, and hopefully have sex with you again and again.

P. P. S. Don't bring flowers or chocolates or gifts on a first date. It's sweet in theory, but ultimately it's overkill and makes your possible new princess feel pressured. Save the gifts for the future. It's the first date, not the prom. She doesn't need a corsage.

Bottom Line: Do what I say and you will land a second date!

Step 6: BE THE BIGGEST BEST DEAL

"I dumped him for the BBD." – One Hot Chick to another

You're doing great so far. I am so proud. You asked her out, she said yes, and you had a good time. Congratulations! Woo Hoo! Hooray for you!

Enjoy the moment.

OK, moment's over. Sorry to break this to you, but just because you had a nice meal and you feel there's some chemistry, you haven't won her over just yet. The fact is a hot woman is always looking for *The BBD: The Bigger Better Deal.* Until you're in a committed relationship— some might say until you put a ring on her finger—you have to compete with every other Joe Schmo that gets up the guts to ask her out. For a Hot Chick to stay with you, decline all other invitations from her many gentleman callers, and commit to being intimate with you, it is essential that you convince her that *you* are the Biggest Best Deal. I'm going to guide you through the crucial courting dates and tell you *how to become The BBD.*

I am assuming you did what you were supposed to do on the first date and asked her for a second date and she said yes. If not, you're looking at starting over with a new girl by going through the steps and finding another first date—and *go get her.* If date number two is indeed on the horizon, this is what you need to do if you want to ride off into the sunset with your lady and live happily ever after… or at least take one step closer to getting her panties off.

Second Date Suggestions

The perfect second date is someplace that you discovered she likes from date number one. It should not just be another dinner but dinner plus something special, like an event. Let's say in talking about music that she mentioned she loves jazz. Great. Plan a date to a restaurant with a live jazz band and dancing or an outdoor jazz concert in the park where you can bring an intimate picnic, or follow a meal with a trip to a sultry jazz bar. Perhaps you talked about how she can't wait to see the Picasso exhibition that just came to town. Find out when she is free and get tickets to the exhibit and pair the outing with a restaurant she mentioned she loves or always wanted to try.

The goal here is to give your Dream Girl *everything her heart desires.*

This can also be your chance to show another side of you. After a romantic, candlelit, gourmet Italian first-date dinner, if you think she's down for it from what you learned about her, go more casual. Let's say she said she's a baseball fan. Fun! Get two *great* seats to a game and suggest hot dogs and beer at the venue in lieu of a sit-down dinner. Perhaps you know that she thinks bowling is totally campy fun and she hasn't been in years. Make a reservation at an upscale alley like Lucky Strike Lanes for a game of ten-pin and bar food. If she said she likes hiking and you know some trails, fill up a backpack with gourmet snacks, a camera, a map, and some chilled drinks and head for the hills. Drawing outside of the typical dinner date lines shows her that you are daring and full of surprises. By choosing things that you know she'll enjoy, you keep her thinking:

"Wow, this guy is really cool. There are a lot of sides to him I like. And, we have so many things in common."

If she is more the opera, champagne, and caviar type, and your wallet agrees with that kind of lifestyle, the second date is your time to show off. Take her to your favorite fine dining restaurant. Order La Grande Dame and the master chef's famous soufflé. If you have tickets to theatre, ballet, or orchestra, break them out and take her on a night of sophisticated pleasures. Prove to her that if she is looking for a life of luxury, she need not look any further than you.

Whatever way you want to go, make sure it is something she will love to do and is available to do it by running it past her first and following the planning and confirming procedure from *"Be a Great Date."* Also, be sure anything you plan is not throwing her into the midst of your close friends, family, or business associates. It is too early for that. This relationship is new and fragile. You need to treat it like the delicate creature it is.

Give Her a Gift

After you give her a welcome kiss, either on her doorstep or your meeting place of choice, the way to a woman's heart is through the gifts you give her. Though diamonds are a girl's best friend, she isn't expecting them on the second date. But know Hot Chicks are used to billionaire businessmen wowing them with glittering trinkets, designer handbags, and luxury label clothing. They have grown accustomed to prolific artists wooing them with songs they wrote about their beauty and paintings they've inspired. You get the picture.

Hot women are spoiled.

Flowers and chocolates, though nice, are not going to bowl us over with their unoriginality. What will win our gratitude, respect, and, therefore, access to our hearts and bodies, are *thoughtful gifts based on you knowing what we like*. You will need to have paid attention during date number one to surprise her with a present on date number two. Get the future love of your life something that you discovered she would want from getting to know her on your initial outing.

For example:

She talked about how much she liked some new *Kings of Leon* song that played on the radio. When you said you've loved them for years then asked her if she knew the rest of their albums, she said no that she didn't. Well... duh. Go make her a mixed CD of their songs from the past ten years or get her an iTunes gift card and make a recommendation list so she can go download their music.

Remember she was goosepimply cold on your first date? You offered her your jacket when you were waiting for the valet because she was shivering. Bring her a Pashmina shawl in a neutral black, beige, or grey so she "will always be warm when she's with you."

Did you two talk about an author, poet, or artist you both love, but she hasn't gotten his or her latest book yet? Go! Get it for her. Come on man, that's your cue.

You don't have to overdo it. You don't have to spend a fortune. You don't want to seem like you're trying to buy her. However, you do want to show her you're paying attention, you're thinking about her, and she's so special you'd go out of your way to get her something unique to her.

Regardless of what you get for her, you must give gifts to your lady out of the goodness of your heart to make her happy. Remember, anything you give her is hers, not yours to take back if things don't work out or she breaks up with you down the road. If you have ever given a woman a valuable item and then asked for it back, it shows you didn't give it in a genuinely loving way. It was really just about you wanting to buy her or make yourself look good. By asking for the gift back, you end up with the opposite effect: looking like a complete asshole. Don't be stupid like Stu in *The Hangover,* who gives the Vegas stripper he just met his grandmother's Holocaust ring.

Don't give it away if you can't part with it for good.

Reveal More of Your Good Stuff

The second date gives you the opportunity to reveal more about yourself and hopefully get to learn more about her. Remember, everything you say should be the happy, positive, cherry-on-top version. If you have any bragging rights to throw around, now is a good time to do it. They don't have to be big things. You just want to give her the idea that you are a successful, likeable guy on the upswing of life. You're the kind of guy she would be lucky to have. Mentioning the good things that you have going on makes her think you're a potential BBD. *For example:*

Let her know that you "just closed a big deal at work" and make a toast to future success.

Mention that you were just "voted president of your condo's homeowners association" and are excited about all of the improvements you're making on the building.

Tell her your "softball team is going to the league championships" and she should come watch for luck.

You just had a complete physical and your doctor said you were "in perfect health."

Everything you say must be truthful, even if slightly sugarcoated for effect. Dating is a lot like selling a used car. You have to point out all the great things so she doesn't notice the dings and scratches. Find some good about you and share it. Avoid complaining about anything or discussing any problems you have in your life. Instead, drop positive little nuggets of information that will plant the seeds of "He's a great guy" in her assessment of you. You may think they're inconsequential, but those little things are the building blocks to you being her *Biggest Best Deal*.

It works like this in her hot babe brain:

You just closed a big deal at work = He is successful.

You're president of the homeowners association = He is popular... and he is a homeowner.

Going to the softball championships = He's a winner.

Doctor's prognosis = He's strong and healthy and, therefore, fuckable.

It's not so hard. Plan in advance some BBD information about yourself that you can work into the second date conversation.

Come Clean Moment

Sometimes it's hard to be honest about certain things in your life, especially ones that she may have a bad reaction to. A come clean moment is a great way to confess something important, and possibly negative about you, while at the same time revealing something positive so she still thinks you're more the BBD for it.

If you really need to get an issue off your chest, start by saying:

"I have something to tell you."

"I have something to tell you" is universal code for brace yourself for bad news. "I have something to tell you" is most often followed with a negative bomb like:

"I'm married"

"I'm an ex-con," or

"I'm a hermaphrodite."

So now, she's prepared for the worst. However, because you are becoming an expert in how to date hot women, you will drop *the bomb* and follow it with a cushion so she'll actually be relived.

For example:

Bomb: *"I've been married."*

Cushion: *"It's been five years now, so I have moved on and am ready for a new relationship."*

Bomb: *"I have a daughter."*

Cushion: *"Her college is paid for in a trust fund I set up."*

Bomb: *"Women have said I'm a workaholic."*

Cushion: *"That's why I make sure to take weekend getaways regularly."*

Promoting the positive side of a potentially negative situation eases tension and leaves her with the impression that even what's supposed to be the bad stuff about you is actually good. Even if there's no big thing to confess, I suggest using the "Come Clean Moment" about something more trivial, though of course true, in your life because it is the best catalyst for your new girl to feel safe to tell you something important about herself in turn. Confessionals oftentimes bring up some red flags and potential deal breakers that are best to know about as soon as possible. What if her response to your "Come Clean Moment" was:

"You were married once so you'll probably understand how complicated it is. I'm separated from my husband. But we still live together."

"You have a daughter. So do I! Well, I did but I lost custody after too many unsuccessful rehabs."

"I'm glad you work a lot. That way I'll never have to."

This is information that is better to know sooner rather than later. It's OK to be direct. If you're not getting anything from her in the form of a confession, it's fine to say, *"So*

I've told you my big secret. Anything I should know about you?" She may not spill the beans right away, but she knows you are open to it when she is ready. It's not meant as a way to get dirt on her as much as it is mean to open the lines of communication to be honest with each other.

Call Her on the Competition

If you have picked up any suspicious behavior that points toward some competition in the BBD department, call her on it. For example, if you notice she keeps getting texts and calls from a caller ID "David" all through your date, it's OK to ask her, *"Who's this David who keeps calling you?"*

If she says "just some guy I used to date," say, *"Why are you taking his calls if he is an ex?"*

Don't back down. Don't be afraid to tell her how you feel. Be the *Biggest Best Deal* of a man by telling it like it is.

For example:

"I really like you. I'd like to see you exclusively. If you are still tied down to someone else, I would rather wait until you're really finished with him."

If she says, *"I really like you too. I've told him to stop calling me."*

Good. Tell her you're happy to pick up the phone next time he calls and let him know she's off the market.

If she says she's still dating other guys and not ready to settle down, don't panic. Tell her: *"OK. But that's not my style. I don't like to share."*

Don't get huffy or possessive. Don't let her see you sweat. Just stay matter-of-fact. Continue on your date knowing you're a great guy with a lot to offer and that she's lucky to have you.

She could be bluffing trying to prove she's in demand. Either way, you're not an insecure boy. You're the BBD. You don't need games or an uncommitted, immature woman. Be cool and follow through. If she says she's still playing the field, don't ask her out on a third date.

Kiss her good-bye and say, *"When you're ready for the real deal, let me know."*

She will probably call you later to tell you she dumped the other dude if you stay strong and don't call her for a week. When she does come back, it will be on your terms.

Tell Her About It

Hopefully there is no one in the shadows, she is totally into you, and you are going to ask her on the third and most crucial date. Don't be afraid to tell her how you feel. *"I really like you. You're a great person"* is not enough. That's what her girlfriend or gay hairdresser says. At this point, on date number two, you need to put yourself out there on the *"Lover Level."* You need to let her know *you are sexually interested in her.* You need to tell her that you *want* her. *"I am really turned on by you"* is what you need to say. Don't be creepy or nasty or start humping her leg like a dog. Simply say something like, *"You are so beautiful. I am really attracted to you."* Keep it simple and she'll think you're sexy.

Manners Are Forever

Don't forget the basic rule of manners of the first date or on the second, third, or tenth date. Open the car door, say please and thank-you, and be nice to service people. Ask her opinion about the menu or what she would like to do. Don't decide for her. Most importantly: *Stay off the phone.* The moment you get on your phone for more than emergencies is the moment she feels you take her for granted. She can then easily choose to be with someone else who will pay full attention to her for at least the length of a dinner. If you need to make a call, excuse yourself, go to the restroom, and do it quickly.

Handy Manly Stuff is Hot

Does your new Dream Girl need a couch moved, a tree trimmed, a sink unclogged, a car fixed, a stereo hooked up, or a computer repaired? Great! Now is your time to show her you are The Man. Now, don't get down on your hands and knees and expose your plumber crack unless you actually know what you are doing under that sink. Making it worse is a total turn-off. However, if you do know what you're doing—bonus points! You may think your tech savvy is a little geeky until it comes in handy with the babes. A girl who can't figure out how to download the latest version of Microsoft Office will be all hot and bothered when you can. Even if you don't have the brains to hook up her Blu-ray to her surround sound or the brawn to do any heavy lifting, you can still be her manly man by calling an audio specialist or moving service you've used and know you can trust to help your lovely lady out of her jam. It tells her you are connected, you can help, and she is lucky to have you.

You to Her Rescue

Now you probably don't have on your Dream Girl list of qualities that you want a woman who is "stalked by her ex", in a "legal dispute" or "is in need of a good dentist to pull an inflamed wisdom tooth." Though these are not good problems to have, they are great opportunities to come to her rescue. Can you help her by confronting a harassing boyfriend to let him know his old flame is newly spoken for? Do you have a good lawyer you can go to for advice and save her some hefty legal fees? Do you have a great pain-free dentist who you can take her to? Be her knight in shining armor by helping her during a time of crisis. Don't get in the middle of anything too messy or dangerous or that you can get sucked into for too much cash. But if you can offer advice, call on a connection or be there to hold her hand through something traumatic; she will forever be grateful to you helping her in a time of crisis and not holding it against her.

Stand Up for Her

I love the scene in the movie *The Fighter* where Mark Wahlberg physically assaults a drunk dude who is hitting on the barmaid girl he likes, played by Amy Adams, and tells him never to disrespect her again. She is, in that moment, totally his. I'm not saying you have to get in a bar brawl to win over a girl. However, you do need to "have her back" if you expect her to consider you her man. When walking down the street, walk on the outside to protect her from passing cars. Hold her hand when maneuvering in a crowd, and make way for her to get through. If you leave to check your phone in the bathroom and come back to find some slimy pick-up artist trying to chat up your girl, step right in and tell him in no uncertain terms that she is taken. Hesitation of waiting for him to leave or making her tell him to get lost is not an option. She is your girl—you must make her feel safe.

Seal the Deal with Something Special

One of the best ways you can assure you are the *Biggest Best Deal* is to bring up something extra special for an upcoming future date. This should be an out-of-the-ordinary event, adventure, or trip that you know she will love and that she can look forward to doing with you in the next month or so. Let's say on your first date you talked about your mutual love of the R & B artist Drake. On the second date, you bring her a mixed CD of your favorite *Drake: Live in Concert* songs. Before the third date, you should find out when he is coming to a city near you and purchase tickets to the concert. When the moment is right, present her with the opportunity. She will be totally excited and say yes to a date with you that may be several weeks or even months in the future. This means she is committed to another several dates with you before then with more chances to grow the relationship and get intimate. This means, she not only likes Drake, she likes you too.

Read the Signs that YOU are the BBD

Once you have successfully shown your babe some reason why you are the BBD, you want to read the signs to see if this girl is really interested in you *sexually*. It's not that hard to figure it out once you know what to look for.

The Hand Hold

When you reach out to touch her hand, does she let you? Or does she pull away? If she pulls away or just merely tolerates for a little while before breaking your hold, she's likely not into you.

If she lets you hold her hand for over a few seconds, it's a good bet she likes to be touched by you.

Even better is if she squeezes it or plays touchy-feely fingers with you.

She is considering you to be the BBD if she wraps her arm around yours and pulls herself in just to get closer to you.

The Little Nibble

If you go in for a whisper in the ear or a light caress on the neck, does she giggle and snuggle back? Or does she turn away?

If she stays close and Eskimo kisses back into your chest, you're in. She is probably getting butterflies in her tummy and wet in her undies.

If she tries to make small talk and pulls back, just know you're not getting into her pants any time soon. You are not yet the BBD.

Initiating Touching

Does your date initiate any touching?

Does she, unprovoked, brush your arm, squeeze your leg, or "inadvertently" rub up against you? If so, you get extra bonus points.

If your little lady takes the lead in the flirty footsie under the table, it is definitely a good sign. She's hot for you. She literally can't take her paws off of you. You're the *Biggest Best Deal*.

Be sure to squeeze, touch, and rub back so she knows you're into her too. She will not continue her advances if you do not respond in kind.

Beware

If she's rubbing up against you and squeezing your leg a little too close to your goods, all the while telling you a sob story about how she's late on her rent because she gave her sick grandmother all her money… so if you could spare just three thousand dollars to get her back on track, she'll do anything…she's not interested, except as the other kind of BBD—The Biggest Best Daddy. Sugar Daddy, that is. She's a con artist/sugar baby who is only interested in your wallet.

Maybe you're OK with that on some level. But really is your BDG (Best Dream Girl) a total user? I doubt: "broke," "desperate," "greedy," or "liar" are qualities you put on your Dream Girl list. Yeah, you may get laid, but it will cost you more than it's worth, and you'll likely only see her again if she needs cash.

Max Out on Making Out

The make-out stage is my favorite part of a budding romance. Saying good-bye with a breathy, lingering, wanting more, good night kiss is so sweetly innocent and restrained. Gently exploring each other's bodies over clothes, like teenagers, gets me so excited. There's something about keeping the mystery alive as long as possible that gets me extremely hot and horny. The angst and anticipation of sex is such a great feeling that you only get at the very beginning of a relationship. So, I believe that it's a shame to rush it. I am definitely no prude. I am not a tease. I love sex! But, keeping the lust alive and not acting on your desires too soon, makes the sex, when it does happen in the not-too-distant future, all the more intense. Holding back and **not pressuring her for sex on the first few dates is the number one way to prove you are the BBD**. You score big points for liking your Dream Girl for more than her body and assuring her that you are interested in a real relationship, not just a one night stand. By staying out of her pants for a few dates, you are way more likely to get in them, again and again.

Bottom Line: Convince her that you are the best guy out there for her so she will want to be with you and only you.

HUDDLE

I'm sure you've heard of *"The Third Date Rule."* This unwritten relationship law states that people must go out on exactly three dates before being formally considered a couple. "The Third Date Rule" suggests that an honorable man does not ask the same woman out on three dates, and a lady does not accept, without the intention of becoming exclusive. Therefore, it is permissible for both parties to partake in sexual activities on The Third Date, as they have passed into relationship territory. At least that's how we women see it. You may simply know the third date as *The Sure Thing*. A third date with this Dream Girl of yours is not just about getting laid. If all you really want is sex, I'm sure you would have chucked this book in the trash by now and been out chasing girls for one-night stands. Don't get me wrong; the magic number could be date number four, five, or even more. But, if it isn't moving forward sexually by number five, it probably isn't going to—ever—unless you are both non-fornication-before-marriage, born again Christians, or some such, and you are both on the same page about not having sex. If that is the case, I'm sorry you have had to read this book so far without being able to enjoy the juicy final chapter to come.

But seriously, every woman and every relationship goes at her, or its, own pace. However, the third date is the first time you should even attempt a move toward sex, if you really want her to know that you are genuinely the *Biggest Best Deal* and that you are serious about *her*... not just getting laid.

Since meaningless sex is not all you're after, the big question for you is:

Are you ready and willing to be in a relationship with this woman?

If you've made it this far, it's more than likely you want to be with your Dream Girl and have mind-blowing sex, not for just one night, but for a long time to come. If that's the case, you'll want to make sure that she's the right girl for you before you commit. Like legendary NBA coach Pat Riley says, *"You want to make the best choice and then go with it."*

Check Your List

Get out your list of your Dream Girl's one hundred qualities. I want you to compare your imagined list to your actual flesh-and-blood live woman. I know you don't know everything about her yet, and that's a good thing. Hopefully, the best is yet to come. However, it's important to take a moment to see if you're on the right track with this one. Just take a look to see what she has that meets your criteria, what she's missing, and what's ultimately important to you.

Twenty or More Dream Girl Qualities

If your *Real Girl* has twenty or more qualities that your *Dream Girl* has on paper, good going, man! You're well on your way. You sure know how to pick 'em. Who would have thought there would be a girl out there with so many things that you want in a woman... who likes *you*. Yes, she likes *you*. She's gone out on two dates with you. She's probably going over her own list right now thinking to herself, *"Wow. This guy's got a lot of the same stuff I was looking for."* Well played!

Ten to Twenty Dream Girl Qualities

Not bad, Mister. Are they physical traits? Personality? Little things? Important things? A mix. Consider this:

What does this girl do or have or look like that you didn't even know you wanted until you met her?

Do you love her laugh, the way she jumps up and down when she gets excited, or the way she hums when she likes her food? Her small hands, her goose bumps on her arms when she's cold, or her come-hither crooked smile? Ask yourself:

What about her would you add to your list of one hundred things your Dream Girl would have that your Real Girl actually has that you didn't even know you would find attractive until you met her? What's she got that you like that you didn't even know you wanted? … Your number may just have gone up.

Under Ten Dream Girl Qualities

Don't give up hope. There's an old saying in real estate: "Buyers are liars." An agent will show a homebuyer, let's call him X, a hundred houses that fit the description of the property he is looking for. He won't like any of them. Then, X will happen to pop in an open house of a place that's completely different than what he and the agent had been looking for, and he loves it! X thought he knew exactly what he wanted, but he really had no idea what would make him happy until he saw it. The same scenario goes for girls. You may say you want:

"A new construction, Italian villa with high ceilings and a big yard"—aka a young twenties, exotic brunette; tall, with big tits.

You go out with eight of this type of woman only to then meet and fall for:

"The restored English Manor with the charming courtyard"—aka a well-kept thirties, fair blond; petite, with a perky ass.

You may have been looking for the wrong woman all along with no luck and then stumble upon the perfect match. Be careful not to toss aside a diamond in the rough. After all, meeting women, getting them to go out with you, and impressing them with your best self is hard work. After some thought, do you still wish your Real Girl had more of your Dream Girl features? Or, do you like your Real Girl better even if she's missing a few because she's *real*.

Can't Find Five Dream Girl Qualities

So she's tall, blond, big-boobed, and well… nothing else. You like to stay home and get up at six a.m. for wheatgrass and jogging. She wants to go out partying every night, sleep 'til four p.m. and start the day with a Red Bull and a cigarette. Or, she needs a diamond and a marriage certificate before sex. You need sex. She wants Prada. Your wallet says nada. If you have some major lifestyle issues, it just most likely will not work. So, move on. After all, you want to be available when your more perfect mate materializes.

Remember: *"You can't always get what you want. But if you try sometimes you just might find you get what you need."* – The Rolling Stones

Step 7: SCORE

Let's Get It On – Marvin Gaye

Congratulations! You've made it to *"The Show."*

Now all you have to do is get some home runs on the scoreboard. Take it from me, Kira Reed, the reporter versed on everything you ever wanted to know about sex, from the erotic to the downright bizarre, a relationship with a Hot Chick is won or lost in the bedroom.

Make It a Sure Thing

Once you decide that you're going to go for it, I am assuming you want to create the best possible scenario for a sexual encounter. If a girl says yes to one of these three dates, she is definitely attracted to you enough to want to have sex with you. Tried and true, *Sure Thing* third dates include the following:

1. Dinner at Your Place

Invite your real life Dream Girl to your house on a weekend night, or night you know you both don't need to be anywhere the next day, for a romantic home-cooked dinner for two. Do not do this unless your place is up to par. A dark, dingy apartment full of action figures will not get you laid. Get rid of any old girlfriend photos, frat boy memorabilia, or anything resembling porn. Your place need not be grand, but organization, a sense of style, and cleanliness are essential. Do not attempt this date if you have roommates, an uncontrollable dog, or anything to hide. Yes, we will look in your medicine cabinet and snoop when you're in the other room. If you can't cook to save your life and you don't have the proper tableware to eat a semi-sophisticated sit-down dinner, leave this to the professionals and order in. Otherwise, you may scare her off. This is the most risky of the three in that there is no reason that she has to sleep over. Though you will get her alone, making out on the couch is a sure bet and can easily lead to carrying her to the bed. Yes, have clean sheets, for God's sake. Be sure to also have a basic toiletry kit, including an extra toothbrush, face cleanser, razor, and moisturizer as well as a set of clean towels ready to hand her if she chooses to grace you with her presence for an overnight stay.

2. A Hotel Rendezvous

This is a bold choice. There is no wiggle room. She cannot get away with *"Oh I didn't realize you wanted sex when you invited me to spend the night at a hotel with you."*

Before you pop the question, check into the availability, rates, and amenities of some of the nicest hotels in your area. This is not a Super-8 kind of date. It's more along the lines of a full-service hotel with in-room dining and a big bathtub for two. A Hot Girl will not be lured by the intrigue of the Holiday Inn. You need an exclusive place with a warm ambiance and an air of luxury. Many hotels offer romance packages that include breakfast in bed or champagne and strawberries upon arrival. You can also BYOB a great bottle of wine. Let her know the wonderful pampering extras you have lined up, like a massage or a room service dinner of her favorite meal. These things will help woo your lady to join you for a night you'll never forget.

3. A Weekend Away

Mark my words: A woman who is remotely interested in you will not say no to a spa weekend at a fabulous resort. If you've got the bank, this is your chance to show her how great life can be with you. Because neither of you will be distracted with work, home, or everyday stress, it's the perfect chance to see how well you are together one-on-one. Don't try this if you have to scrimp on the place. Only go for it if you're going to go first class. Most anything by the seaside or lakeside is fabulously relaxing and really feels like a vacation. Make sure your destination of choice is adults-only or at least has areas like an adults-only pool so you're not forced out of the mood by screaming kids. Spa treatments are a way to a woman's heart. So, be sure to indulge your lovely lady with some rubbies and scrubbies. Just think of it as foreplay—she does. Also, be certain there are several restaurant choices and leisure activities nearby, like movies, art galleries, and shopping so you aren't stuck for things to do in between lovemaking sessions inspired by your sexy resort weekend.

I have to say, as a hot-blooded woman who enjoys sex that "The Third Date Rule" really does hold true for most women I know. A truly hot woman doesn't throw herself in bed with just anyone. She likes to know what's in man's head before she finds out what's in his pants. After all, the largest sex organ we have is the brain. It's one thing if you're dating a young girl who is a virgin or some nonsense like that. Otherwise, if the sophisticated lady that you've been wining and dining says yes to one of the above-listed three dates, she likes you and thinks you have promise based on the previous two dates she's had with you. Now that she has gotten to know you as a person, she wants to see what you're like in the sack. If you're looking to have an amazing first sexual encounter, just do what I say and you will succeed.

Sex Soundtrack

Whether you're cuddling up with your sweetie at home or whisking her off to a weekend away, your seduction scene must have a soundtrack. It is a great idea to create a mix of twenty or more of your favorite songs to make a playlist for sex. Everyone has different musical tastes, so it's hard to advise exactly what to include on it. However, I've come up with a few no-fail tips.

Instrumental mixes like St. -Germain or a favorite ambient groove album are good ideas if you don't want to be lyrically bogged down. If you're more into whatever is on the Top Forty hits mix, and you know she is as well (because you've talked about it on one of your previous dates), you can go that way. Just don't get too edgy or genre-specific unless you know she's into it, i.e., you don't want to bust out the hardcore gangsta rap unless you know she's down. If you're a Frank Sinatra and Nat King Cole kinda guy, make sure she is too before you lull her to sleep with your "oldies" music. Or, play it safe by updating the classic sounds with the more contemporary artists like Diana Krall, Harry Connick Jr., or Michael Bublé. If you're not sure what will get that dress off her back and onto the floor, tried and true timeless rock classics and sexy pop favorites are a good bet. To give you an idea, one of my sex soundtracks lists reads like this:

"Here Comes My Girl" *Tom Petty and The Heartbreakers*

"Let's Get It On" *Marvin Gaye*

"With or Without You" *U2*

"Rock With You" *Michael Jackson*

"Every Breath You Take" *The Police*

"Angel" *Massive Attack*

"Lovers Rock" *Sade*

"Use Somebody" *Kings Of Leon*

"Just Like A Woman" *Bob Dylan*

"Crazy For You" *Madonna*

"Romeo and Juliet" *Dire Straits*

"Chasing Cars" *Snow Patrol*

"Tiny Dancer" *Elton John*

"Time After Time" *Cyndi Lauper*

"All Night Thing" *Temple Of The Dog*

"Crash Into Me" *Dave Matthews Band*

"Breathe In Breathe Out" *Mat Kearney*

"Wonderful Tonight" *Eric Clapton*

"In Your Eyes" *Peter Gabriel*

"You Make Loving Fun" *Fleetwood Mac*

"Dance All Night" *Ryan Adams*

"Seems Fair" *Several Hundred People*

"Come Back To Bed" *John Mayer*

"Maybe I'm Amazed" *Paul McCartney Wings*

Best Bet

Pick something you know you both like because it's been a topic of conversation on a previous date. For example, maybe you bonded over dinner on your last date that you both went the same Killers concert back in the day, before you had met... blah blah blah... and wished that you had known each other then. Playing some Brandon Flowers and Killers tunes will surely get her ready for lovin' because it brings you closer together, reminding your Dream Girl of your wonderful compatibility and mutual interests. It will remind her of your unique common ground and your charming ongoing attentiveness. Let's say you both, surprisingly, have a penchant for disco era Diana Ross because on a previous night out, to your utter disbelief, you both sang the words to a verse of "Love Hangover" and then both giggled in embarrassment because you thought you were the only ones in the world who liked that song! Put that on the playlist for sure to reiterate your destined-to-be-together-ness! Music is a powerful tool that can be used to your advantage.

No Clue What to Do?

Confused as to what will get her hot and bothered? If you're not sure what will rock her world, allow me to recommend Sade, as I have never known a woman who doesn't love her. *Love Deluxe*, *Lover's Rock*, and *The Best of Sade* are all fantastic sex soundtracks. Most women will need to change their panties by the second verse of any one of her songs. You can play the entire albums from start to finish and there are no take-you-out-of-the-moment tracks.

Of course, you can also simply ask what she would like to listen to.

No-Nos

My advice to you is to leave out the over-the-top love stuff. For example, I have the following songs on my iTunes, but I wouldn't necessarily put them on my third-date sex soundtrack:

"Just the Way You Are" *Billy Joel*

"When a Man Loves a Woman" *Percy Sledge*

"Have I Told You Lately" *Rod Stewart*

The above love epics are indeed romantic; however, they are too heavy-duty for a third date. Keep it cool and save the super-sappy stuff for the third *anniversary* mix. You don't want to scare her off with too much too soon.

DO NOT, under any circumstances, include cheesy songs like the following:

"The Wind Beneath My Wings" *Bette Midler*

"My Heart Will Go On" *Celine Dion*

"I Will Always Love You" *Whitney Houston*

Also, skip anything by Liza Minnelli, music from a Broadway show, or anything mashed-up by the cast of *Glee*. Your Dream Girl will most likely run for the hills, never to return because she will simply assume you're gay.

Lotions, Potions, Candles, and Such

I know, you're a guy and you don't necessarily need scented massage creams and edible love oils to get you excited for sex. If you're like most men, all you need is a visual of some cleavage and you're good to go. However, we ladies like soft-skin-making, pretty smelling, delicately tingling lotions, potions, candles, and such. So, it is essential that you have them on hand to guarantee the success of your *sure thing*.

If you are at a loss as to what to get because your knowledge of fragrance is limited to deodorant and aftershave, then you may need some assistance. You probably have a neighborhood "pleasure store" or a little perfumery in your area. Great. Go there, tell the sales girl you are planning a special sexy evening, and have her show you the goods.

You can't go wrong with Kama Sutra products that are available at many specialty stores. I've featured them in my Playboy TV shows because I am totally in love with them. Kama Sutra uses the highest quality ingredients and the most delicious scents, including their "Classic Bedside Box," which includes *The Original Oil of Love, French Vanilla Body Soufflé, Love Liquid Sensual Lubricant,* and

Sweet Honeysuckle Honey Dust with feather applicator that serves as a great starter package. You can also get their "Weekender Kit" that has travel-size versions of their favorite yum-yums if you are taking your lovely on a sexy score getaway. I have tried almost everything on the market and Kama Sutra products are indeed my favorite. Check them out at Hustler, on the Sunset Strip, if you're in Los Angeles, or in any other love shop, wherever you may be. Don't forget ordering online if no other opportunity exists.

If you are planning on having your girl over to your bachelor pad, then you should know that candles are the key toward a perfect night. They create a soft, warm glow that makes women want to cuddle up. Candlelight, and dim lighting in general, makes most women less self-conscious, more at ease about their appearance, and, thus, more likely to want to get freaky. Many candles have a perfumed scent, which can serve as a nice aphrodisiac. Just be sure it's a natural fragrance so it's not too overpowering. I especially like gardenia, lavender, citrus, and vanilla. However, I only burn one scent at a time as to not overdo it. Candles in glass jars are the best because they won't make a waxy mess when they melt and they contain the flame for safety. Avoid the Glade-like plastic odor control candles and sprays you find at grocery and drug stores. Those are fine for behind your toilet to eliminate everyday man stink; however, they are mostly synthetically scented and not special enough for a Hot Chick. VOLUSPA makes Dream

Girl- *worthy* candles that are available at most upscale specialty shops. Be aware that hotels frown on candles due to fire hazards so leave them at home. Be sure to watch the flames while you're rolling around in the moments of passion because burning your Dream Girl's hair off will totally ruin the moment.

Libations

A little wine is fine and can help both of you get in the mood. I recommend a nice bottle of white or whatever cocktail you've learned she likes. If you're not sure what to serve, try champagne and strawberries. I know it sounds a bit cliché, but clichés become clichés for a reason: because they work. Just be careful not to overdo it out of nerves. She'll just get sloppy and you may become too numb to get it up. You don't want to blow this very important first sexual encounter by being too plastered to enjoy the moment. You don't get any points on the scoreboard if you're too drunk to remember hitting the home run.

Condoms

You must buy them. You must bring them. You must use them. Unless you are one hundred percent hunky dory with your new woman being pregnant after date three, you have to wear a condom. I have had several friends stupidly attempt the "pull out method" and get preggers. I know *Knocked Up* was a cute movie, and Katherine Heigl is one hot momma who's totally out of Seth Rogen's league;

however, unprotected sex rarely leads to a happy ending—no pun intended. Do not try it. Be a good boy and wear your raincoat. I don't mean to scare you (actually I do), but I have seen smart, savvy, single guys trapped into being baby-daddies before they are ready and willing. Their seemingly sweet girlfriend said she was on the pill, but she really wasn't. She just wanted a baby and/or child support and/or to keep the guy around. Most women are honest and loving and would never betray you. Then again, there are the Oksana Grigorievas of the world, so just remember: only you can prevent baby bumps!

Though I don't particularly enjoy being a nag and playing the role of remedial heath class teacher (I do like to role-play teacher-student now and again), there are these very real things called STDs. For those of you who skipped class to go smoke pot under the bleachers, sexually transmitted diseases are nasty, painful, puss-filled, and, most importantly, they can be fatal. You don't want to get one and you don't want to give one. It totally sucks that something that feels so good can make your dick feel like it's being burned alive. But STDs, including AIDS, are life-and-death serious shit that totally take the fun out of riding bareback. Just surrender to the fact that condoms are required until you check off on each other's blood test results *and* you are in a mutually monogamous relationship.

One of the reasons why guys hate wearing condoms is that they miss the slickness of the vagina. Lucky for you, God invented lube. When you pick up your ten-pack of condoms, be sure to grab a lubricant as well. I like Astroglide, KY Liquid, and Eros, to name a few. Just be sure that whatever you get is condom- and latex-safe, which will be clearly labeled on the package for you. OK, no more lecture. I'm not a doctor and I've never even played one on TV, so I will stop with the condom talk. Just please be safe and sane and wear them, or I will have to say, "I told you so!"

The Five Things You Must Do

OK, now for the juicy stuff. She's agreed to meet you at your place or the hotel you've planned or to travel with you to a weekend getaway. You're in! It's a sure thing because you've followed the steps up to this point and you've set the scene for romance at your rendezvous spot of choice. Turn on the tunes, dim the lights, and chill the wine. The ball is in your capable hands now, and it's time to score. Here are the five things you *must* do to get from standing in the middle of the room dressed to sprawled out naked in bed with your Hot Babe.

1. Perfect the Art of Kissing

Kissing is the most intimate form of connecting to a person and the gateway to every other aspect of sexuality. If you are a bad kisser, chances are you won't get past first base. In order to not mess up this most important act, I offer this advice: *once you make lip-on-lip contact, let her take the lead.* The way she kisses you will inform you how she likes to be kissed. Does she smooch and separate, softly nip, or run her tongue over your lips? Feel what she does and then reciprocate.

To win the game of kissing, leave her wanting more. Hot Girls are so used to men not being able to control themselves; it will help your chances of getting in her pants if you don't rush to jam your tongue down her throat. Most women will agree that forceful tongue thrusting should be saved for deep, passionate lovemaking. I cannot tell you how many times I have been turned off by the way a man practically killed me with a kiss. A too sloppy, overly exploratory, sucking face kiss is not sexy—it's assault. Trust me, if you kiss like you're trying to win a tonsil hockey contest, your date will fake food poisoning just to get away from you. Remember, your Dream Girl is a delicate creature and you don't want to hurt her.

Allow the gentle kissing on the mouth to lead to kissing down her neck and light nibbling on her ears. The nape of the neck and earlobes are usually very sensitive areas. Even soft blowing on these places will send chills down her spine and make her want you to make the next move. However, you don't want to give her a Wet-Willy because it's just plain gross.

Be sure you're not a *Dirty Bird* with scratchy stubble or bad breath. A smooth, freshly shaved face and brushed teeth are essential prerequisites for the perfect third date smooch fest and all other subsequent encounters. Shave the five o'clock shadow right before the date, if possible, to be extra soft for her. Have mouthwash and/or mints and dental floss on hand as well. Believe me, onion breath and spinach in your teeth is not hot.

2. Caress Her Whole Body

A woman's body is one big erogenous zone. It's not segregated into just two parts: tits and ass. If you want to steal home base, don't rush to the second base boob grope or third base crotch grab before you spend some time in the outfield—otherwise known as *foreplay*. Gently caress her shoulders, arms, hands, thighs, etc. Going straight for a breast before she's warmed up is a very amateur move reminiscent of awkward encounters in the seventh grade. To get her ready to go all the way, explore everything *else* first before the typical go-to goods. Here are some places you may not think a woman would want attention that will win you points toward your ultimate goal.

Her Stomach

Many women find kissing, biting, and light tickling on their stomachs erotically pleasurable. It can cause strong arousal—almost as strong as stimulation of the genitals—lucky them! I particularly like soft blowing on and light licking of my belly button. Every woman is different, so pay attention to her responses to see what is working for her.

The Inside of Her Arms

The skin on a woman's arms, armpits, and especially the inner arms is highly sensitive to stimulation. Light stroking with your fingers or gentle kisses on the inner arm can initiate arousal down below. The middle arm at the bend of the elbow is super-sensitive due to the area's thinner skin, which makes nerve endings more accessible. Try giving her little kisses from her wrist to this sweet spot. It is a sensual sensation that totally gets girls wet.

Her Fingers

The fingertips have many nerves and are sensually responsive to stroking, sucking, and playful biting. The sides of the finger can be ticklish too. Both light and firmer touches work well on the fingers. I love a tiny bit of tongue between my fingers. It gives me butterflies—everywhere.

Her Feet

Due to the concentration of nerve endings in the soles of the feet and toes, the sensations produced by caressing the feet can be extremely pleasurable. I love getting my feet rubbed. In fact, I don't know a woman who doesn't. I also love having my toes sucked. Not only is it great foreplay having my toes sucked, stroked, and licked during intercourse (yes, I am very flexible), it also totally intensifies my orgasm.

3. Make Her Feel Beautiful

Another thing you must do to guarantee a great score, is *tell your Dream Girl how beautiful she is.* Believe it or not, hot women are insecure about their bodies just like everyone else, especially when undressing in front of someone for the first time. Because their identity is so tied to their looks, most beautiful women, even more so than average-looking girls, need to be told how gorgeous they are in order to feel comfortable getting naked for you. As you start to take each other's clothes off in the natural progression of kissing and caressing, tell her how unbelievable she looks as you go.

As you slip her shirt gently over her head to reveal a pretty, lacy bra with overflowing cleavage, don't rush to rip it off. Look at her body, gently moving your fingers over her curves, her shoulders, breasts, and waist. Describe to her what you see and how it makes you feel, like:

"Your skin is so soft. I love touching you."

"Your legs are so strong. I can't help stroking them."

"Your stomach is so tight. You're making me hard."

Again, it's not just about her tits and ass because you're not just giving her general lip service but making complimentary observations about her beauty. Whisper in her ear how you can't wait to see her naked because she is the most gorgeous woman you have ever seen. Though it seems superfluous to point out her obvious beauty, you must tell her how hot she is to assure she's naked in your arms and totally uninhibited in bed.

I know there is some inane, screwed up mind fuck theory out there promoted in "How-To-Get-Laid" books like *The Game* that claim that, in order to get a girl to sleep with you, you have to make her feel unworthy and, therefore, grateful to have you, with thinly disguised jabs and backhanded insults, like, *"Your stretch marks really aren't so bad."* Let me be clear here: if you tell your about-to-be-bedmate that she's *"pretty good looking for a woman her age"* or she would have *"an incredible body if she just lost five pounds,"* you will not score. You will get slapped. The make-her-feel-bad-about-herself nonsense does the exact opposite of its supposed intent. It's COMPLETE BULLSHIT. If you make a girl feel ugly, self-conscious, or unworthy, you will surely be left with blue balls...and likely a black eye.

Unless you are looking to screw low self-esteem, pathetic, scared little girls that will likely turn out to be man-hating nutcases, insults will not get you laid. Only genuine compliments will win over any girl worth winning over.

4. Go Down Good

I'm sorry to break it to you, but your almighty cock will only get you so far. I've kicked many a man to the curb in my day for not performing oral sex. Take it from me, if you say, *"That's not my thing"* or *"I don't need to eat pussy because I have a big dick"* you will not be welcomed back to her bed. If you want to please your Dream Girl, you have to go down on her. I'm not talking about little teasing sissy licks... I'm talking about full-on devouring her pussy until she comes-all-over-your-face cunnilingus. This is not negotiable. I don't care if you've had bad experiences in the past with a woman who doesn't like it because she's frigid or afraid of intimacy. It doesn't matter if you have been turned off by some girl somewhere along the line who didn't know how to groom or wash properly. Get over it! Your Dream Girl is a modern, sexually advanced woman who loves a good PL (Pussy Licking) and knows how to take care of herself. So, you shouldn't have any fishy issues down there.

If, for some reason you are not into it—get into it! Do you think women innately just can't get enough cock down their throat? No. We give blowjobs for *you*. We like it, and do it, because it makes *you* feel good. That's what is pleasurable to us: pleasing you. Going down on her pleases her; therefore, it pleases you—end of story. If you aren't blessed with absolutely loving it, like my man (lucky me), don't even hint to her that it is a chore. She will be self-conscious about it and *not enjoy having sex with you*. It is your job to give your woman satisfaction in bed. If you don't, she will likely go elsewhere to get it.

Remember the scene from *When Harry Met Sally*? Any girl can fake an orgasm. To make sure she's really getting off, you have to go down. Here are some basics:

The clitoris is the visible button-like thingy above the opening of the vagina. It is basically the female version of your penis. This is the part of your Dream Girl you must stimulate in order for her to orgasm.

- Don't forget to shave. Scratchy scruff hurts those lips too!

- It is called "eating pussy" not "tasting pussy." Get a mouth full of clit and enjoy.

- Take your time. You've worked so hard to get here, where else do you have to go?

- Little quick licks can be annoying. Deep, long sucks are orgasmic.

- Tongue first. Fingers second. To be pleasurable, she needs to be slippery before you slip anything in.

- Get into the groove. Follow her reactions to find a rhythm...then stick to it. If it ain't broke, don't fix it. You don't want to stop what you're doing if you can hear and feel that she is really enjoying what you are doing.

- Let her take control. As the pleasure builds toward orgasm, she will likely steer her hips and clit in the exact direction, force, and speed she needs to reach climax.

Because no two women are alike, it's hard to give exact instructions. For me, the biggest turn-on is enthusiasm. Though you can explore various licks and sucks and pressure to find what your lady likes, don't get too hung up on specific technique. Also be vocal. It's OK to ask,

"Does that feel good?" Sometimes, by no fault of your own, but because a woman's orgasm is elusive and stems more from her brain more than anything else, no matter what you do, it's not going to do it for her. Or other times she may not be in the mood for a PL and just wants a good hard fucking; thus, by all means, just give her what she wants. However, on a first sex date you *must* attempt to go down on her so she knows you are ready and willing for when she does want it. Have no fear about being good at it. As long as you're down there, a woman will guide you and grind into you to make it feel amazing for her. Then, once she explodes in pleasure through clitoral stimulation, your Dream Girl will be dying to return the favor with an enthusiastic blowjob and want to continue her orgasmic bliss by fucking your brains out. So go down on her. It is a win-win for everyone!

5. Fuck Like a Porn Star

In all the years I spent interviewing adult film stars, sex experts, and erotic icons as a reporter for *Sexcetera,* I found that all great sex has one thing in common: you must *mix up positions!* You don't have to master the *Kama Sutra,* own a closet full of sex toys, or break out the ropes and chains. However, you do need to change up your sexual configurations to keep it interesting. I mean, when was the last time you watched a porn scene that was all one position? You haven't because they don't exist! The rule on any adult movie set is that each scene must have at least five positions. Take it from the professionals: you need to let go and let it *flow*.

Not only does mixing up positions keep the lovemaking lively, it also helps you prolong orgasm because you're taking a breather in between set-ups. In fact, changing positions is what the male porn stars do if they feel they are about to cum before their cue. It's a good idea, if you feel you're climaxing too soon, to switch it up.

Here are some shape-shifting ideas:

Master Missionary

I don't know why plain ole *missionary* (she's on her back, you're on top) gets a bad rap for being boring. It is a great place to start and really get a feel for each other. It's the best position to enter and establish a solid rhythm before getting more adventurous. I personally find missionary to be the most romantic and intimate of positions because it's face-to-face, breath-to-breath, lips-to-lips. Going for something too complex right from the beginning, especially with a new partner, can be disastrous. You must find out how you fit together in the basics before getting more advanced. Besides, you don't need the pressure of mastering a *pile driver-corkscrew* right off the bat. Missionary does not mean just pounding away at her like she's a blow-up doll. Use this starting position to explore her body. Caress her hips and cradle her breasts with your hands. Stroke her hair. Look into her eyes and connect. Then, to extend the experience and make sure she isn't just laying back wishing you'd get it over with already, you must flow from missionary into other positions. For example:

Drive Her Legs

Moving up on your knees, pull one of her legs up over your shoulders and you'll be able to give her a nice deep thrust. This is a great angle for adding in any toe sucking and foot play and gives her the chance to take more of you in. You can then spread her legs into a wide "V" position on either side of your head, steering them gently like the wheel of a car to "drive" into her. Be careful not to get too crazy stretching her in all directions like Gumby before knowing how bendy she is. This is a fun variation of the basic man-on-top that most anyone can do. Even the prissiest of "pillow queens" will be pleased with this pole position because you are doing most of the work, so she can concentrate on moving to get maximum pleasure for herself, which of course feels amazing to you too!

Flip Her Sideways

Turning your lovely lady on her side can really help you get a whole new feeling. "Flipping" her is the perfect way to get full access to her body. When she's on her side, front, and back, breasts, tummy, hips, and ass are in reach, which really gives you something to hold on to. It's a very fluid position that reaches the inner and outer areas of her vagina for variations of stimulation. You can gently rock her back and forth to find the right spot for both of you. It's OK to talk and ask her how she likes it. A little *"How does that feel, baby?"* and *"Ooh, God, that feels good. How about you?"* keeps the juices flowing.

Do Her Doggie

I love getting a good banging from behind. *"Doggie"* style is a dominant position for the man but also gives the woman sturdy leverage to thrust back into him so she can really go for it. Be gentle to begin with, especially if you have a very large or curved penis. Let her move back and forth on her hands and knees into you harder and harder as she gets wetter and wetter. In the doggie position, your girl can easily reach back with one hand to stimulate her clit or play with your balls at the same time you're thrusting into her to heighten the intensity. This is a great position to try a little light spanking and gentle hair pulling to add some edge and get the blood flowing to all the right places. Just remember to not overdo it until you know her better and know what gets her hot …and what does not.

Up Dog/Down Dog

Once your girl is on her hands and knees grinding into you, you can change it up a bit by pulling her to the edge of the bed and standing up on the floor behind her. In this doggie variation, you can spread your legs wide over her ass and have her press her knees tighter together, snugger around your penis, as you continue to thrust. This is a great position to take charge of the motion and angle by guiding her hips. You can also control the pace to make sure you don't pop if you're not quite ready and want to try another configuration. From *Up Dog*, you can press her butt *down* so she's lying flat as you thrust her while keeping her legs squeezed together. It's a nice tight hold around your cock and brings the friction to the more shallow, outer region of her vagina for a whole new kind of sensation. Ass men love these alternate doggie styles, and your girl will be impressed as you take control and seamlessly lead her from one position into another. Just be careful not to crush her in your enthusiasm, big guy!

69

To 69 or not to 69? That is the question. I see a lot of showy "69" positions in porn films with tongues all stretched out in a show for the camera. I get it in theory; however, in reality I can't really relax and get off on what you're doing to me while I'm busy doing the same to you. And unlike in the movies, it's not tongues out that do the job; rather, it is mouth-on devouring. So, with both of you going at each other it can sometimes get suffocating. Don't get me wrong, I love getting a good PL and giving blowjobs. However, 69 can be a little too much multitasking and I'd rather enjoy giving or receiving separately rather than all together. But, that's just me. I do think "69" is good for warming up and getting the party started or mixing in to change up the stimulation to prolong orgasm.

Ride 'em Cowgirl

Rolling her on top will give you a break from being the aggressor and give her a chance to take charge. Perched on penis, she can ride you just how she likes it. This position is always used in erotic movies because it is a great position to show off the girl's body. In real life, it's great for you to be the "audience." As she arches her back, she will stick her butt out and protrude her breasts forward. She'll flip her hair and rhythmically move to your sex soundtrack playing in the background. You get to lay back, relax, and enjoy the show. It's good to be you. Having her on top may also help teach you what she likes because she is setting the tone and rhythm, while being in the saddle.

Reverse Cowgirl

If you're lucky, your Dream Girl will pretend your shaft is a sit-n-spin and swing around for a little Reverse Cowgirl action, or you can guide her in that direction. Yes, it feels as good as it looks. Be sure you are nice and hard before you move her on top because you need to be a strong horse for your "cowgirl" to ride. It is also a super-intense sensory overload position, so don't go to it too fast. You're likely to blow your load quickly, and you don't want to buck her off before she gets a good ride.

Screw Her to the Wall

If you've got the strength, picking her up and balling her against a wall can be totally hot. Women love a big strong man who can carry her out of bed and across the room. Just don't forget a wall is hard, so no slamming in the heat of passion. You don't have to hold her up the whole time; instead, simply place her on a high chair. A barstool can be easier on your back while still offering new angles of action. Don't forget the dresser and table and the floor while you're at it. Just remember to grab a blanket or pillow for some comfortable padding.

Back to Basics

If, after all this banging, you're still in the game, it's nice to come back to basics. Roll back into some variation of missionary. Take a moment to connect and look into your Dream Girl's eyes. Gently breathe her in, kiss her, and acknowledge how much you like her and enjoy being with her by telling her:

"You are beautiful."

"You are amazing."

"You make me feel so good."

"I didn't know it could be this great."

"I love making love to you."

(Skip the "I love you" statement until the sober, dressed light of day, or you might regret it. Saying it in the throes of ecstasy is too easy. Once it's out there…it's out there.)

When it comes to scoring with your Dream Girl, whatever you do, don't try to map out the sex too specifically. Making a list like: *Go down on her for five minutes, then start with missionary for two minutes before moving on to doggie style for one minute ...* will not lead to mind-blowing orgasms. It will result in cold, calculated, boring, boinking. Sex is a basic human instinct and is supposed to be fun. It's not an exact science to be taken too seriously. Everybody is different and every woman likes to be kissed, touched, and made love to in her own distinct way. So don't overthink it because it's more about surrendering to the moment, reading her reactions, and not worrying so much if you're doing it right. *Don't think. Just fuck.* If you ask me, sex is eighty percent enthusiasm and twenty percent technique. One of the main reasons why adult stars like Jenna Jameson, Sasha Grey, Jessica Drake, Tori Black, Evan Stone, and Sean Michaels are so erotic and powerful to watch is that they love sex and go for it with boundless enthusiasm. The porn kings and queens thoroughly enjoy giving and receiving pleasure. As the star of your own sex life, so must you.

Erection Issues

Unless you have serious issues that you are seeing a doctor about and your penis performs like Gary Dell'Abate pitches, skip the Viagra and other erection-enhancing drugs. Please don't recreationally pop little blue pills. It's a myth that women want to fuck forever. We don't want you to have a hard-on lasting six hours. It's just too much! If you come rather quickly, don't get insecure. Your girl will actually feel good about it if you turn it into a positive. Tell her that she was "so hot you couldn't control yourself." She will likely be forgiving and feel special that she turned you on so incredibly much. Give her a killer PL, then wait for a while, or the next time you see her (after all, Dream Girls aren't a one-shot deal), go for it again. You are bound to have more stamina and be more confident the second or third time around.

The only thing we hot women *really* don't like to do is spend three hours trying to get your dick up and running to no avail. So help us out. If you know what works for you, tell her, show her, or do it yourself while she strokes your chest or caresses your balls. If you like your ass tickled or right nipple pinched or her feet in your mouth, tell her. Because you have already satisfied her with a great pussy licking, she will most likely be perfectly happy to accommodate most all of your desires.

Fetishes

Being a Playboy TV reporter for seven years was the best sex education I could have ever hoped for. Some of my experiences were erotic, many were surprising, but mostly they were a bit bizarre. One of the things about the show that I am most proud of is that we always attempted to demystify perversions and find a way to understand and relate to people's fetishes. We tried never to label people as *"weird"* or *"wrong."* We simply asked the question: *"why?"*—"why does someone lust after the things they do?" Uncovering the answers of what drives desire and what creates a particular fascination was my favorite part of my job. As an embedded reporter in the sexual underworld, I loved putting myself in other people's shoes… or latex, or body paint, or pony gear, or ropes, or chains, or clothes pins, or chocolate sauce, or...whatever excited them. I was turned on by being able to walk the line between journalist and participant and, every once in a while, cross nine toes over it. Ultimately, what I learned is that there is a fetish for *everything*. And, if you think you are alone in what gets you off, you're wrong. There is nothing that isn't a turn-on to someone, and if you are into something "bizarre," don't worry—there is some Hot Chick somewhere in the world that is into it too.

However, at least at the beginning of a relationship, avoid getting *too into* what you're into. Don't go nuts with the hair pulling, plastic wrapping, erotic asphyxiating, dressing up like Iron Man, or whatever it is you do out of the mainstream-ordinary on the first visit to the bedroom. If you really need a fetish fix to get even remotely excited, try going for a little taste of it. If you like to be dominant, attempt a light tap on her ass to see if she's responsive. However, don't overdo it the first time out. A little spanking goes a long way for someone who doesn't include it in her own sexual repertoire. Let's say you have a *"trample"* fetish. You may scare her off if you ask her to walk across your chest and stomp on your balls with her high heels. However if you simply say, *"I like it when you leave your shoes on,"* she may enjoy wearing her sexy stilettos to bed. You can then slowly, over time, work in some more advanced scenarios for your mutual enjoyment. Save the heavy machinery like restraints, nipple clamps, double-ended dildos, whips, chains, and milking devices for future dates—and only introduce her to your deviant practices after you've discussed your mutual interests. Hopefully, she will find some level of eroticism in your interests as well, especially if you can help her understand *why* it is you like it.

Note: If you are a heavy into practicing anything—BDSM, swinging, exhibitionism, etc.—you may want to go to AdultFriendFinder.com or other alternative lifestyle websites or clubs to meet your Dream Girl. The fetish that you have is likely as important to you, or more so, than the sex act itself. So your need to have her be excited about your fetish must be on your *Perfect Woman List* from the beginning if you are going to find your right match. Remember, the average, run-of-the mill Hot Chick will not want to be tied up and ball-gagged, order you to lick her boots, or get you off by having sex with other people in front of you. So if a specific fetish is what you want, you may need to venture out of the average, run-of-the mill places to pick up girls.

Build Your Sex Toy Box

Though you don't want to whip out your vibrating bullets, beads, and balls on your first *sure thing* and scare her off, it is good to be prepared for anything, including dates four, five, six...and so on. I recommend building a *Sex Toy Box*. There are few essential "sex-cessories" that everyone should have on hand besides condoms and lube. They are a *vibrator*, *a blindfold,* and *padded handcuffs.*

I live in Los Angeles and there are plenty of places to unabashedly shop for sex toys, from the mega-store Hustler of Hollywood to the ultra-chic Coco de Mer. I'm sure you have a sex shop in your hometown as well, but if not, sex toys are what mail order and the Internet were invented for. No matter where you live, I recommend visiting California Exotic Novelties (calexotics.com). I produced a show about the company for Playboy and was lucky enough to be sent home with three lifetime supplies of sex-enhancing devices of all shapes and sizes. Needless to say, my Secret Santa gifts that year were all the rage. The Cal Exotics name is synonymous with great quality adult toys, and there is definitely something for everyone. Check them out to get:

A Vibrator

When choosing a vibrator that both you and your Dream Girl can enjoy together, my advice is to stay away from realistic (cock-looking) devices. That's what we have you for. We don't need a stand-in. Go for something pretty and fun like purple, clear, or metallic. A vibrator is not meant to replace you but to add to your roster of ways you can please your lady. I don't know any woman who doesn't enjoy a nice vibrating wand of some sort now and again for a change of pace. Some of my tried and true favorites include *The Jack Rabbit and The Magic Wand* and handheld varieties by Dr. Laura Berman, like the *Danae*. When in doubt, get several shapes and sizes.

A Blindfold

A blindfold is one of the most versatile items that can be used for sex play. I mean, what woman doesn't get excited recalling the Mickey Rourke/Kim Basinger blindfolded-by-the-refrigerator-covered-in-honey scene from *9½ Weeks*. Keep your lover in the dark with a silky, lined blindfold available at most pleasure stores. Or, you can make one with a scarf or even her stockings. Just slip something over her eyes and take control of her sense of sight, which, in turn, will heighten all of her other senses.

Padded Handcuffs

Get your bondage on in a soft and sexy way by restraining her with some fur-lined or leather cuffs. They will offer a smooth, pleasurable feeling while maintaining a sexy sense of constraint. Look for the kind that has an attached ring, which allows you to connect the cuffs to the bed or any other furniture. Be sure they are padded so they don't cut her wrists, but stick to black color in case you want to play up your dark, sinister side. It's hard to pull off a damsel in distress scenario with pink, furry cuffs.

You should also include in your *Sex Toy Box* any costume or accessories that transform you or her into someone or something that turns you on, like a stethoscope to play doctor, thigh-high stockings, cat o'nine tails, latex gloves … or whatever floats your boat. However, skip the blow-up dolls and molded porn star pussies. Your Dream Girl won't appreciate the competition.

All the accessories aside, if you *perfect the art of kissing, caress her whole body, tell her how beautiful she is, go down good,* and *mix up positions,* you will score enough points to win the girl of your dreams again and again. So, save some of the kinkier stuff and secret stash of goodies for keeping future dates fresh.

Further Afield

Of course, once you score, you will want to do it more and more. That's why I produced *69 Sexy Things 2 Do Before You Die* for Playboy TV. We included simple, sexy, stay-cations and sensual getaways, guaranteed to keep things hot for you and your girl.

Some of my favorite segments include:

Create an Ultimate Bubble Bath with Sensual Bath Products by KamaSutra.com

Have 101 Nights of Great Sex LauraCorn.com

Honeymoon "Without Getting Married" to Costa Rica
RanchoPacifico.com

Make Love Under The Northern Lights of Alaska
ChenaHotSprings.com

Take A Trip To Tantalizing Tulum MayaTulum.com

We also did some fetish vacations and ultimate swingers events. You can see more about them all at

www.playboytv.com/shows/69-Sexy-Things-2-Do-Before-You-Die

So many sexy things to do... so little time! But stand warned. I want to offer a word of advice.

I do not recommend swinging to you and your new girl.

If that is what you discover works for you both, or if you both are already in the "lifestyle," great! You will find Swing Fest on your own. However, in a new relationship that is still developing, or any relationship, no matter how solid you feel it is, bringing multiple partners into your sex life can be devastating. If you want your budding love to last, I recommend sticking to the sweet stuff you can do together.

Bottom Line: You've got her. Get it on good!

LAST WORDS

I sincerely hope this book is a help to you. Though the goal is to SCORE, there are several possible scenarios for the outcome of this book. All of them are positive.

1. **WIN**

    CONGRATULATIONS! Woo Hoo! Double back handspring into side-kick splits!

    Mission accomplished. You got your Dream Girl and you will live happily ever after. Hopefully, you'll keep discovering that your new real life girlfriend embodies more and more of the important things on your Dream Girl list, like *"She is an expert in the cheerleader-seduces-nerd role-play scenario."* SCORE!

2. **PLACE**

    Let's say you make it through all the steps, get a girl to go out with you, and then it doesn't work out. Bummer, dude. It happens to the best of men. The good news is, you know the system works because you did indeed win a girl…just not the right one. It may be time to refine your list of Dream Girl qualities. What are some of the attributes you thought you wanted in your lady but then they didn't turn out to be such turn-ons after all? A change of goal can lead to a change of result.

3.   SHOW

I am so proud of you. You showed up and gave it your best shot. Now we just need to refine your game. Where is your scoring potential puttering out? Is it in your personal presentation? Finding a girl? Getting her to go out with you? Closing the deal by proving you are the BBD? You need to determine where it is in the steps you are losing your stride so you know what it is you need to resolve. Then reread those sections and get back up on that horse.

One of my favorite quotes of all time is Winston Churchill's *"Never, never never, never, give up."* I always forget how many *nevers* he actually said, but we get the point: NEVER. Remember, failure is always great practice for success. All the practice you've had so far in meeting and dating women is valuable experience necessary to close the deal on your next Dream Girl.

One More Thing to Remember

Once you win your woman, don't get lazy.

Treat your lady with the same respect and attention on the one hundredth date as you did on the first. Don't take her for granted. After all, she's *yours* and therefore special.

Please know that a hot woman is powerful, independent, and sought after. She's not a little doll you can dress up and boss around. She's a force to be reckoned with, a delicate flower to protect, and a sex goddess to be worshipped— all wrapped into one amazing package. To keep the romance passionate, treat your lady like the goddess that she is. Regular praise for her beauty, intelligence, and individuality is necessary. Words and shows of affection beyond, but including, throwing her down on the bed, are key. Keep small gifts and romantic date nights in your repertoire. Listening to what she says and what she likes and accepting who she is does not end after you get laid. Scoring is just the beginning of your ongoing efforts to make and keep her interested and happy.

Your Dream Girl may be irrational, emotional, and chameleon-like at times. You may call it crazy, and that's fine by me. Women are complicated and everyone is a little nuts in their own way—including you. No one is perfect. Thank God! Perfection is too hard to live up to.

Although there are plenty of fish in the sea, they're all slippery little suckers and can easily get away. Stay diligent in your quest to be the best man you can be and make her feel she's the only woman for you. After all, you've worked hard to get her. Don't let her go.

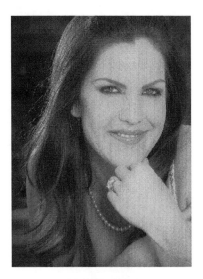

ABOUT KIRA

Kira Reed is an actress, television host, writer, and producer. After graduating UCLA's School of Theatre Film and Television, she enjoyed a prolific on-camera career including a seven–year stint as a reporter for Playboy TV's *Sexcetera.* Kira was the writer and supervising producer of the travel reality series *69 Sexy Things 2 Do Before You Die* and is currently an entertainment reporter for Associated Television International and the spokesperson for MyMedicalRecords.com. She lives in Los Angeles with her husband Bob Lorsch and their menagerie of rescue animals. See more of Kira @ KiraReed.com.

All photographs by Christopher Robert Burke

Made in the USA
Charleston, SC
15 December 2012